The Pain-Free Back

THE
Pain-Free
Back

**6 SIMPLE STEPS
TO END PAIN
AND RECLAIM
YOUR ACTIVE LIFE**

Harris H. McIlwain, M.D.,
and Debra Fulghum Bruce, Ph.D.

AN OWL BOOK

HENRY HOLT AND COMPANY · NEW YORK

Henry Holt and Company, LLC
Publishers since 1866
115 West 18th Street
New York, New York 10011

Henry Holt® is a registered trademark
of Henry Holt and Company, LLC.

Library of Congress Cataloging-in-Publication Data

McIlwain, Harris H.
    The pain-free back : 6 simple steps to end pain and reclaim
your active life / Harris H. McIlwain, and Debra Fulghum Bruce.
        p. cm.
    Includes bibliographical references and index.
    ISBN 0-8050-7326-4
    1. Back care and hygiene—Popular works.   2. Backache—
Treatment—Popular works.   I. Bruce, Debra Fulghum, 1951–   II. Title.

RD771.B217M424 2004
617.5'64—dc22   2003056936

Henry Holt books are available for special promotions
and premiums. For details contact: Director, Special Markets.

First Edition 2004

Designed by Victoria Hartman

Printed in the United States of America
1   3   5   7   9   10   8   6   4   2

To Linda and Bob

Contents

Introduction

As a rheumatologist and pain specialist, I wrote this book to help improve the health of your back. Knowing that back pain affects four out of five adults at some point in their lifetime, I want to give you everything you need to know about back pain—its causes, its cures, and, most important, how to prevent it.

In this book, I want to show you how taking care of yourself right now will help you have a stronger back and a healthier life in general. I want you to recognize lifestyle behaviors that may put you at risk for back problems and learn how to change those behaviors. I want you to have a better understanding of medical tests doctors use to diagnose back pain and the latest medications that may give you fast relief. If you are suffering from back pain right now, this program will show you how to take control of your life and resolve this pain so you can be active, feel great, and even keep the pain from coming back again.

A Painful Problem

Back pain is a condition that crosses age boundaries, affecting as many young adults as it does adults over age fifty-five. Even though older adults get back pain from osteoarthritis, osteoporosis (thinning bones), or disk disease, America's current emphasis on sports and fitness results in many younger adults getting back pain because of injury, overuse, or exercising improperly.

Most of us know what back pain feels like, especially weekend warriors after they've spent a day playing tennis or golf, biking, or even doing yard work. Next to the common cold, back pain is the most common reason people visit their doctors. In fact, in the United States, back pain is

- The most prevalent cause of disability in men and women under forty-five
- The nation's number one occupational hazard
- The third most frequent reason for surgical procedures

Each year back pain results in more lost days from work than any other ailment except arthritis and related diseases. Of the $27 billion spent on all musculoskeletal injuries annually, $16 billion is spent in the management of lower back pain; more than half of that $16 billion is spent on surgical treatment.

Assessing Your Pain

I know it's difficult to think of pain as a positive sign, but it is. Pain is your body's natural signal that there is a potential problem. Without this warning, you might cause irreparable injury. While this feeling is the body's way of alerting the brain that there's a problem, when back pain continues for weeks to months, it becomes a part of your entire being and existence. At that point, not only is the back pain a symptom that something is amiss, but pain becomes the disease itself.

What Causes It?

When my patients talk about back pain, most of them are usually referring to the most common type: lower back pain in the lumbar spine. It is estimated that 70 to 90 percent of back pain is caused by muscle, tendon, or ligament problems, usually along with weakness in the lower back. Nevertheless, sometimes back pain can affect other parts of the back, including the upper and middle back, and it can radiate down the legs to the feet (called sciatica).

Many structures in the lower back can cause pain, including the muscles, ligaments, tendons, bones, small joints in the spine and disks. Some of the most common causes of back pain include the following:

- Osteoarthritis due to deteriorating cartilage
- Injuries or accidents resulting in muscle pain
- Osteoporosis due to bone loss and fracture

- Fibromyalgia with tender "trigger points"
- Serious diseases such as cancer in the spine and organs

More serious forms of back pain can cause numbness in the legs, hands, fingers, and even loss of bladder and bowel control.

Acute or Chronic?
Back pain can be acute or chronic, depending on the problem and amount of tissue damage.

Acute pain is sudden and severe. Most of the time, acute pain is a symptom of an injury or diseased tissue. In more than 80 percent of cases, acute pain goes away in about two weeks; it runs its course and disappears as the problem is relieved. If your back pain from a strained muscle lasts only a few days or weeks, it is considered acute.

Chronic pain lasts more than three months or longer. With chronic pain, our bodies react differently. Instead of serving a protective function like acute pain, chronic pain continues to send messages to the brain through the nerves even though there is no tissue damage. When pain becomes chronic, you might have brain hormone abnormalities, low energy, mood disorders, muscle pain, and impaired mental and physical performance. Chronic pain worsens as neurochemical changes in the body increase your sensitivity to pain and you begin to have pain in other parts of the body that do not normally hurt.

Chronic or long-term pain affects sleep for weeks to months, even years, causing you to awaken frequently at night and experience daytime sleepiness. This long-term back pain can cause appetite loss, muscle weakness, irritability, and depression. You might have difficulty dealing with others, including family members, friends, and people at work.

Unlike acute pain, which is a sign of a healthy nervous system, chronic pain takes on its own life and mimics a disease. When pain persists for weeks or even months, it can cause an increase in the level of cortisol, the body's main stress-induced hormone. Although the immune system needs a certain amount of cortisol, when it becomes elevated for an extended period, it can impair the cells that make up your immune system and overall function.

Because of being bathed in the stress-related chemicals, the immune system can find it harder to function optionally. Living with unending chronic pain and the subsequent stress, your immune system simply will not work at full capacity. This breakdown in immune function can interfere with your ability to keep infections at bay, long-term healing, and quality of life. New studies indicate pain might affect the immune system in such a way that it speeds the growth of cancer cells.

When to Call the Doctor
If your back pain happens for the first time, then it is reasonable to ask your doctor for advice to diagnose the problem. If the pain lasts for more than a few days, then it is even more important to seek help, as the pain can interfere with your work and activities. However, pain that is severe and unending should alert you to seek immediate medical evaluation. Call your doctor if any of the following symptoms occur:

- Pain that is worse with a cough or sneeze
- Back pain or numbness that travels down one or both legs
- Pain that awakens you from sleep
- Difficulty passing urine or having a bowel movement
- Loss of bladder or bowel control
- Weight loss
- Fever
- Pain in another bone or in the abdomen

These problems may be the earliest signs of serious nerve damage or other serious medical problem, such as arthritis, osteoporosis, cancer or diseases of internal organs, and need early treatment for the best results. (Before you begin your *Pain-Free Back Program*, review the chart on page xv.)

There Is a Solution

No matter what causes your back pain, this common condition can be easily treated and prevented with specific lifestyle measures. *The Pain-Free Back* is the result of my passion to teach men and women how to have healthy backs using a simple, 6-step holistic program. I call it a "program" because that's exactly what it does—it *programs* you to have healthy back habits for life.

In writing this book, I'm not only interested in the condition of your back. I want you to become healthier as a whole person—in your mind and entire body. For instance, if you are sedentary, you might need to start a regular exercise program (Step 1), which will strengthen the key

Do you have back pain with numbness or pain extending down the leg?	➤ You may have a ruptured (herniated) disk (see page 178).	➤ Talk to your doctor for a diagnosis.
Do you have back pain and sudden loss of bladder or bowel control, or weakness in a leg?	➤ You may have a more serious complication of a herniated disk (see page 179).	➤ Emergency! If you have lost bladder or bowel control, call your doctor. Go to an emergency room to be seen immediately.
Does the pain stay in your lower back and become worse with twisting and bending?	➤ Your pain may be from a muscle spasm, a pulled muscle, or a compressed nerve (see page 173).	➤ Talk to your doctor if the pain does not improve after a week.
Did your back pain start suddenly with bending or lifting or falling? Are you also over age sixty?	➤ You might have a fracture in the spine.	➤ See your doctor. Treatment is available for pain and to prevent future fractures.
Do you have a fever along with back pain?	➤ You might have a serious infection (see page 181).	➤ See your doctor.
Do you have blood in your urine and one-sided back pain along with burning during urination?	➤ Your symptoms may be from a kidney infection, or kidney stones (see page 181).	➤ See your doctor.
Do you have a blistering rash and burning pain on your chest or on your back and down one leg?	➤ Your pain may be from a viral infection called shingles.	➤ See your doctor.
Do you have back pain with stiffness in the morning or other joint pain or swelling?	➤ You may have ankylosing spondylitis. This is a form of arthritis that affects the lower back. Other forms of arthritis can also cause back pain (see page 180).	➤ Call your doctor. To relieve pain, use the 6 steps in the *Pain-Free Back* Program.
Do you have back pain during pregnancy?	➤ Pregnancy causes stretching of the ligaments around the uterus and pressure on the lower back.	➤ Consult your doctor if the pain continues or if fever or bleeding accompanies the pain.
Is the pain centered in the lower spine? Do you have pain radiating down your leg to your knee or ankle?	➤ You may have a ruptured or herniated disk (see page 178).	➤ Consult your doctor.

muscles that support your back and abdomen, and benefit your body and mind as well. If you are overweight, not only will that increase your chance for back pain and injury, it puts you at higher risk for chronic illness, such as hypertension, heart disease, diabetes, and cancer.

My Pain-Free Back Healthy Eating Plan (Step 2) will help you get back in control of what you put into your body so you can get down to a normal weight, ease pain, and feel more energetic. Knowing that stress is a key player in back pain, in Step 5 you will learn better ways to deal with stress, which if left unmanaged can take its toll on your overall health. In each step of my program, I'll help you to recognize unhealthy lifestyle behaviors and replace them with healthy ones that will possibly eliminate your back problem forever.

In the past three decades of helping men and women with back pain, I've learned a lot. Now, through my *Pain-Free Back Program*, I want to help as many of you as I can to recognize the true cause of your back pain and teach you how to be proactive in preventing it. I want you to see how improving the health of your back will improve the health of your entire body. I want you to be able to recognize the signs and symptoms that result in back pain and to know what to do if you become affected—*before* you suffer serious problems. I also want you to ask for the proper medical treatments for relief, if and when you need them.

How This Book Can Help

This book is based on my professional belief that the approach each of us takes toward preventing and treating back pain must be custom-tailored to our individual lives and situations. With each of the 6 steps, I will help you to understand your personal risk of back pain, so you can take the necessary actions to reduce that risk—and enjoy an active life longer. Among the many things you'll learn in the *Pain-Free Back Program* are

- How exercise is the gold standard for strengthening your back and the specific exercises that can ease pain within days
- How the right diet and nutrients can decrease inflammation, ease pain, and help you to get back to a normal weight again
- How to sit, stand, bend, lift, and carry loads so that you don't suffer a back injury
- How the computer workstation may be the cause of many back problems and what you can do to make it ergonomically correct

- How mind-body therapies can help reduce daily stress and ease back pain as well
- How natural dietary supplements play a role in healing your back
- Which special situations might need medical attention, such as osteoarthritis, osteoporosis, and disk disease
- Which of the latest medications stop inflammation and pain, so you can get back on your feet again

I've had too many busy men and women tell me over the years that they really don't want a detailed explanation of back pain—the intricate and often confusing medical reasons of why they feel the way they do. Rather, they want to know how to resolve it quickly. As you read this book, you'll see how page after page of personalized self-care strategies can be used immediately to stop back pain in its tracks. I want you to get *fast relief,* and my 6-step program will help you do just that!

6 Natural Steps to End Pain

Here are the 6 steps I will present in the *Pain-Free Back Program:*

Step 1: The Pain-Free Back Exercise Program. This step will show you which types of exercise restore strength, improve posture, and alleviate pain and disability. You can get great relief within days of starting the specific stretching, conditioning, and strengthening activities described here. Of all the steps, the exercise program is vital.

Step 2: The Pain-Free Back Healthy Eating Plan. Being at your ideal weight is necessary to resolve most types of back pain. Step 2 introduces ways to make healthy eating choices that result in easing you back to a normal weight, which will alleviate your pain.

Step 3: Back to Nature. In this step, you'll learn how to use complementary and alternative medicine (CAM), such as natural dietary supplements, poultices, rubs, and salves, among others, to relieve pain.

Step 4: Back to Basics. Making key lifestyle changes will help you live pain-free. This step instructs you in how to sit properly, stand without slumping, how to lift heavy items and carry kids and grocery bags. I also explain how on-the-job tension may increase your risk for back pain—

even though you aren't involved in heavy physical work—and what you can do to reduce this risk.

Step 5: The Pain-Free Back Relaxation Therapies. Stress plays a big role in back pain, but there are ways you can counteract the daily stress of career, commitments, and an "out of control" life. This step helps you sort through your main stressors and provides you with enjoyable mind-body exercises that will change your response to stress.

Step 6: Healing Touch Therapies. A host of touch therapies are known to ease back pain—massage, structural alignment bodywork, chiropractic, acupuncture, and acupressure, among many. Step 6 will explain how these treatments work and assist you in finding the therapies that are best for your type of back pain.

Here's to Your Health!

I realize each person who reads this book is different, and your prevention or treatment program must reflect your individuality. For instance, some of you have two or more problems that can result in back pain, such as osteoporosis and osteoarthritis. Or you might have an old back injury from high school days, along with fibromyalgia or other type of arthritis. Sometimes pregnancy can result in a painful back, and it's important to know what measures you can take that will not harm the unborn baby. Whatever back problem you have, I hope to address it in this book and help you regain control of the pain—and your life.

In more than twenty-five years of practicing medicine, I have learned a lot about treating back pain. My goal is to help you understand ways to prevent and treat back pain using lifestyle measures to keep your back healthy. Your goal is to change the behaviors you can control so that you greatly reduce the chance of having any more problems. After all, you only get one back for life, so you had better take care of it!

Now, let's get started.

PART I

Your Pain-Free Back Program

6 Simple Steps to End Back Pain and Reclaim Your Active Life

The Pain-Free Back
Exercise Program

When I first met Sandy Michaels, she had suffered from back pain for more than a decade. This forty-year-old software designer and mother of two had resorted to working at home because she could no longer endure the painful thirty-minute drive to her office. Each time her car stopped in traffic, Sandy experienced shooting pains throughout her back. Sitting at the computer workstation was painful, too, and Sandy was afraid she would need surgery, which is why she came in for an evaluation.

As we talked about her medical history, Sandy said that she had tried almost everything to resolve her back pain—from acupuncture, massage, and heat packs to herbal therapies, homeopathy, and even biofeedback. Nothing seemed to help. Even the strong narcotics her former doctor had prescribed were ineffective after she took them for a while. And the drugs made Sandy so exhausted she could not work or take care of her young children.

When I asked how often she exercised, Sandy was quick to respond, "Not at all." She explained her fear of injuring her back even more and that she was very guarded in all her movements to avoid more pain. "And, besides," she added, "I blame exercise for my back pain, as I was first injured when I fell playing softball ten years ago."

Even though Sandy had such negative feelings about exercise, I convinced her that moving around with increased activity was the best way—the only way—to help her to feel relief. Exercise would allow her to reclaim her active life again—a life without debilitating back pain and immobility. Sandy started the Pain-Free Back Exercise Program, which

> ## Start Your Pain-Free Back Diary
>
> Using an inexpensive three-ringed notebook or PDA (Personal Data Assistant), you will keep a daily Pain-Free Back Diary throughout the 6 steps in this program. For Step 1, use the diary to record your daily exercises, including the type of exercise (stretching, strengthening, and conditioning), the time of day, the duration, and how you felt before, during, and after exercise. Also, write down how you feel after using the moist heat or ice applications on your back before and after exercise. Take your Pain-Free Back Diary (or PDA) to your next doctor's visit, and review the feelings and any concerns you have experienced during and after exercise. Talk about exercise restrictions, if any, and ask if medications might help you to stay pain-free.

you'll learn about in this step, and within three weeks she surprised herself with much less pain and greater mobility.

After two months on the *Pain-Free Back Program*, Sandy told me she was sleeping better, taking less medication, and had gone back to work at her office, giving her the much-needed social contact she was missing while working at home. She even joined the Y and started a regular water exercise program to keep her back strong—and pain-free.

Sandy is just one of more than 100 million adult Americans who experience some degree of lower back pain each day. According to a new survey by the American Academy of Physical Medicine and Rehabilitation, more than half of those people say that back pain interferes with their daily activities. Ironically, of those who complained of back problems, only a small percentage said they have gone to a medical doctor for a proper diagnosis and treatment. In addition, while almost half of those surveyed believe surgery is the only answer to their problem, in reality surgery is needed in only about 5 percent of back pain cases.

Exercise and Your Back

If you are like most of my patients with back pain, you are tired of hurting and probably cringe when the word *exercise* is mentioned. Maybe you identify with my patient Kim, a young woman who injured her back during a step-aerobics workout. Even though Kim was a passionate athlete, she developed a real phobia about exercise, fearing she'd reinjure her back again. Kim reasoned that if it hurt when she moved her back doing stretches, and it was not as painful when she didn't, then being less active would help to resolve the problem. Wrong!

Or, perhaps you're like forty-eight-year-old Mac, a high school science teacher, whose back pain occurred when he bent down to pick a paper clip off the floor. Overweight and underfit, Mac swore off exercise for months for fear that the slightest motion would cause his back to go out again. "After all, if picking up a paper clip could cause this much pain and loss of work," he said, "imagine what regular strength training or stretching might do."

When back pain patients like Kim and Mac come to our clinic, the first recommendation I make is, "Exercise." I explain that in almost every situation, whether with injury or degenerative disease, most cases of back pain can be reduced—and even stopped completely—with regular physical activity. Stretching, strengthening, and conditioning exercises can result in stronger muscles that support your spine and your body's weight. And when your body's skeleton is supported, you are less likely to suffer injury and pain. A number of excellent studies show that when back pain sufferers start a regular exercise program, including resistance exercise or strength training, they are more likely to have *less pain*, return to work, and be active again. These men and women are also less likely to need as much medical care for back problems if they continue to exercise. I like to tell my patients that if they start the regular Pain-Free Back Exercise Program, the chances are great that instead of making another trip to the doctor for more tests or medications, they'll soon be on the golf course or tennis court actively enjoying their lives.

The Cycle of Chronic Back Pain

When most people get back pain, they become less active. Many patients immediately go to bed for days, hoping to resolve the pain. They sit around instead of moving more and avoid using their muscles as much as possible. Because of this, the muscles that bolster the spinal column weaken. After avoiding exercise for weeks, the back can lose muscle tone and strength, feel tense or tight without any movement, and even begin to feel achy or hurt more for no reason at all.

Many times this never-ending pain causes less and less activity. Decreased activity causes more discouragement, which in turn can lead to sadness or depression. Depression results in further decrease in activities. The more inactive you become, the less you will exercise, and the more likely it is that pain will increase. As you will see, much of the *Pain-Free Back Program* is directed at these parts of the cycle.

Treatment of back pain is important, and the earlier treatment begins, the better the chances of improvement. This means that the effort and treatment applied during the early stages of back pain can give *better results* than the same amount of treatment and effort later on.

Pain ⟶
  Decreased Activity ⟶
    Discouragement ⟶
      Depression ⟶
        Less Activity ⟶
          Increased Back Pain

Figure 1.1

Cycle of Pain

Move More . . . Not Less!

Miranda had just recovered from a back injury sustained in a car accident when she reinjured herself doing a simple household task. This thirty-six-year-old mother of three was lifting her son's backpack out of her car when she felt a sharp knifelike pain in her lower back. As she slowly walked to her house, she wondered how this could have happened again. After all, she had intentionally avoided lifting or any physical activity that might increase pain or cause injury.

Most people with back pain do try hard to avoid using injured muscles—and that's probably the biggest mistake they can make in healing. In doing so, they rely on extra muscles in the back, putting far more strain on their backs than normal. The more muscles they use, the greater the load on the spine. In fact, slowly lifting even a light object, like a bag of groceries or child's backpack, increases the time that the spine has to bear the extra force. For Miranda—and for millions of back pain sufferers—there is a tremendous need for education in how to prevent back pain altogether by moving more, not less.

Bye-Bye, Bed Rest!

Kerri worked in our administrative office for several years. This forty-six-year-old bookkeeper was slim, active, and extremely fit, until she fell while skiing in Vermont. After her fall, which fractured two vertebrae, Kerri ignored the Pain-Free Back "rules" and literally went to bed, hoping rest would help her heal. When a week in bed did nothing to resolve the pain and only made her feel weak, Kerri took a three-month leave from work; she would call in periodically to say she just could not move because of the pain. Within a period of three months, Kerri gained more than twenty pounds from this sedentary lifestyle, her back pain worsened, and she lost a lot of muscle strength in the lower back and legs.

It was once thought that bed rest was the ultimate cure-all for back pain. As recently as a few years ago, patients with back pain were told to go to bed until they felt strong enough to walk around. Even when they were mobile again, patients were instructed to minimize their activities to avoid further injury—exercise was not part of the treatment or prevention program at that time.

Today we know differently. While a very short period of bed rest may help reduce acute pain, we know that for *every week* of bed rest, it may take *two weeks* to rehabilitate the patient. Studies show that patients with back pain who continue their daily living activities have better back flexibility than those who are confined to the bed or a sedentary recovery. *Flexibility* means the ability to move your back through its full range of motion.

Fifty-year-old Jim is a believer in exercise as a cure-all for his chronic back pain. Just before undergoing spinal repair surgery for a herniated disk, Jim decided to try exercise. As a CPA, Jim was extremely sedentary and was about forty pounds overweight, so not only would exercise help to strengthen the muscles in his back, it would also help him lose weight—another back pain remedy.

Jim started the 35-minute exercise program recommended in this step and said he finished four minutes the first morning and then quit. When I spoke to him on the phone, I urged him to stay on his pain medications and use moist heat applications before and after exercise to alleviate pain, reduce muscle spasms, and decrease inflammation. I also challenged him to increase to five minutes the next morning. When I didn't hear from Jim for about six weeks, I wondered if he had given up entirely or changed physicians because he didn't like this remedy.

Pain-Free Back Suggestion

Limit bed rest to one day at the most, and start exercise immediately, even walking around your bedroom, your house or apartment, or your yard. Gradually increase exercise, as you are able, and then begin the Pain-Free Back Exercise Program as your pain decreases.

Jim finally called my office and said he was doing the 35-minute workout daily, and his pain had resolved a great deal. He was feeling better, had lost eight pounds, and felt as if the best decision he'd ever made was when he opted out of surgery. It's been a year since Jim started his Pain-Free Back Exercise Program. Today, he has completely recovered from his painful bout of back pain, and he continues to exercise daily, using a combination of strengthening or resistance exercise, twice-daily stretches, and swimming laps in his pool.

5 Ways Exercise Stops Back Pain

I realize that it's difficult to comprehend how increasing activity will give you great benefits in pain relief, especially if your back has been hurting for a while and keeps you from performing normal daily activities. Still, if done on a regular basis, physical activity and exercise will *relieve your back pain* and strengthen the muscles that support your back. In fact, sometimes medication should be the last consideration for long-term treatment for back pain. Exercises, along with weight loss and important lifestyle changes, are often most important in helping you to stay active. Once you stop moving around, your back problems—and pain—may escalate. Let's look at five ways exercise will help you end back pain once and for all.

1. Strong Muscles Give Support to the Back
Regular exercise such as walking, swimming, resistance exercises, stretching, or yoga helps to reduce back strain, improve posture and range of motion, and strengthen the muscles that support the back. Exercise can also prevent osteoporosis (which results in painful fractures), help maintain mobility, and prevent falls—another risk factor for back pain.

When you train a muscle to work over its full range of motion, it will remember being stressed under those conditions and work efficiently when you need to lift or carry an object, play recreational sports, or simply get through your day more efficiently—without pain. However, if you strengthen the muscle in a limited range, or ignore it and avoid exercise altogether, you will greatly limit the muscle's function, which can easily lead to injury—and chronic pain.

2. Strong Abdominal Muscles Improve Posture
Strong abs help to improve posture and overall balance, and support the lower back. More than simply standing up straight, good posture means using your body correctly at all times—when standing, sitting, sleeping, and exercising.

3. Increased Flexibility Aids in Movement
When your body is toned and flexible, you are less likely to get off-balance or fall, which can result in injury. When muscles are used, they become increasingly shortened. As you stretch and move the muscles through their full range of motion, you will counteract this shortening and keep muscles flexible. Improved flexibility also prevents abnormal force on the joints and helps to decrease injury.

4. Stronger Bones Prevent Fractures
Exercise strengthens your bones. Weight-bearing exercises—such as walking, jogging, jumping rope, climbing stairs, tennis, and resistance workouts—are all crucial to increasing bone mass and preventing osteoporosis.

5. Exercise Boosts Natural Painkillers in the Body
Exercise boosts the body's production of endorphins, pain-fighting molecules that may also be the reason for the well-known "runner's high." Endorphins also help to reduce anxiety, stress, and depression. Studies show that exercise helps restore the body's neurochemical balance and triggers a positive emotional state.

Exercise and Specific Concerns

I will discuss each of the following specific back problems in detail in Part II, "Special Situations." It's important to recognize that exercise is beneficial for almost all back problems.

Disk Disease

Disks are small cushions that separate the bony spinal vertebrae. You might think of your disks as being like small shock absorbers for the spine. Wear and tear on a disk can cause it to become ruptured (or herniated), resulting in a gradual or sudden break in the supportive ligaments surrounding the disks in the neck or lower spine, especially between the fourth and fifth lumbar vertebrae. A disk might become herniated because of a sudden injury or stress on it, such as obesity or improper lifting. The risk of having a ruptured disk increases with having to constantly lift heavy objects or poor fitness habits. Once the disk ruptures or herniates, the disk material causes inflammation, pressure on the spinal nerves, and results in tremendous pain.

Exercise helps those with disk disease by strengthening the muscles that support the spine and the tissues around the spine. If you start exercise gradually and slowly, increasing from a few repetitions to the full Pain-Free Back Exercise Program, chances are you will be one of the 90 percent who will not need surgery because of disk disease. With new evidence that spinal surgery is not the cure-all for most people, exercise should become widely recognized as the ultimate therapy that works for the long haul to keep backs strong. And it's free!

The spine is made up of a column of bones (each one is called a vertebra). There are a total of 33 vertebrae in five sections:

1. The cervical spine (the neck)
2. The thoracic spine (the middle part of the back)
3. The lumbar spine (the lower back)
4. The sacrum
5. The coccyx

Each vertebra is named according to its section and its number from the top—C1 through C7, T1 through T12, L1 through L5, and the sacrum-coccyx section, which are formed into one and are not movable.

There is a disk between every two vertebrae, which acts as a cushion or shock absorber for the spine. The disk has a strong outer layer of cartilage and a soft inner portion. When a disk ruptures, the soft inner portion expands into the area around the disk, which can cause inflammation and pain and may cause pressure on a nerve.

The disks act as strong connections between vertebrae. Joints on each

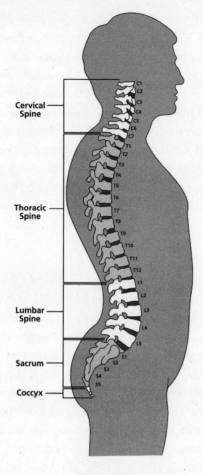

Figure 1.2

The Spine

side join part of one vertebra to the next. These joints help movements of the spine. There are several ligaments, which are strong bands that connect the vertebral bones, attaching one vertebra to the next. Tendons attach muscles to the bones.

Arthritis

Exercise increases range of motion and decreases pain for those with arthritis. Osteoarthritis (OA), also known as the "wear-and-tear" type of arthritis, is the most common form of arthritis and usually affects those who are over age fifty or who have an injured joint such as an athletic injury of the knee. The cartilage, which usually cushions the joint, becomes worn and less efficient. Osteoarthritis is most common in the joints that bear the weight of the body—the knees, hips, and spine—and in joints that have been injured. Osteoarthritis usually comes on gradually over the years and is more common in those who are overweight.

For those with OA in the spine, exercise is the most important part of treatment. If started slowly with only a few repetitions at first and then gradually increasing, as you are able, exercise will increase your muscle strength to give the spine more support. Exercise also increases the flexibility of the spine and the muscles around the spine so you can move easily and smoothly.

Osteoporosis

Exercise keeps bones strong and helps to prevent fractures for those with osteoporosis. Osteoporosis, or thinning of the bones, can result in fractures, pain, surgery, and disability. While other back problems may have early warning signs, osteoporosis is often not detected until a fracture happens. In women, the total amount of bone present may peak from age 25 to 30 (or even earlier in some women). Then the tide turns. At some point, usually around 35, women begin to lose bone, sometimes at a rate of 1 percent per year. This rate increases to about 4 percent per year during the five to ten years after menopause (usually age 45 to 55).

With men, bone loss can happen, too. In fact, about 30 percent of osteoporosis patients are men. Although this disabling problem may start ten or more years later than with women, osteoporosis can be just as disabling and painful. Osteoporosis can be detected early—before fractures—with a simple bone-density test (see page 171). With a bone-density test you don't have to have that first fracture!

Weight-bearing exercises stimulate the cells that make new bone. By increasing weight-bearing exercises, we encourage our bodies to form more bone and delay or actually reverse the destructive process of osteoporosis that results in painful or debilitating fractures. By adding strength training, you improve your muscle strength, flexibility, and reduce the likelihood of falling, as you get older. One-third of all women who live to age ninety may break a hip because of osteoporosis, and men are vulnerable, too. I believe that daily exercise is a small price to pay to keep bones strong and fracture-free.

Types of Exercise

As you start your Pain-Free Back Exercise Program, I want you to focus on the three types of exercise that follow.

Stretching Exercises

Almost all patients with back pain can get great benefit from daily stretching of the connective, or soft, tissues—the muscles, ligaments, and tendons—around the spine. Your back, including the spinal column and its adjoining tissues, is intended to be in motion. Any restrictions in movement can actually worsen the pain you feel and set you up for injury.

When we have sedentary jobs, work at the computer for hours on end, or avoid exercise because we're simply lazy, our once-flexible muscles shorten and become less supple. It's not the actual muscle fibers that limit our range of motion. Rather, it's the connective tissues and the involuntary action of our bodies. There are three types of connective tissue:

1. *Tendons*, which connect your muscles to bones
2. *Ligaments*, which bind bone to bone inside the joint capsules
3. *Muscle fascia*, which makes up as much as 30 percent of a muscle's total mass and is responsible for about 41 percent of a muscle's total resistance to movement. Many of the benefits we get from stretching, such as joint lubrication, improved healing, better circulation, and enhanced mobility, are related to the healthy stimulation of fascia. It is one tissue you can stretch safely.

Stretching increases flexibility. Studies show that stretching helps increase the muscle's elasticity and can increase how long and hard you exercise. This flexibility is determined by several factors, including:

- The intensity and types of physical activity performed
- Gender (women are more flexible than men)
- Age (flexibility will decrease with age if you don't stretch)
- Temperature (warm muscles are more flexible than cold ones)

Stretching boosts healing. Regular stretching lengthens the muscle tissue, improves blood flow throughout the body, and speeds the essential delivery of oxygen and other key nutrients to your back. Usually, when you have an injured or aching back, you will also have some progressive stiffness involved. A regular stretching program allows you to gently push your range of motion to help mobilize the spine and soft tissues for continuous pain relief. Your stretching exercises should focus on achieving flexibility in the spine, muscles, ligaments, and tendons, as well as muscles not directly involved with the back area such as the legs and arms.

Stretching prevents muscle strain and soreness. As you do your Pain-Free Back stretches regularly, you will notice that it becomes easier to move your body, to reach for items on high shelves, or to bend down and look for something under a desk. Walking becomes easier, and your sense of balance will get better, too.

Pain-Free Back Stretching Strategies
To start: The Pain-Free Back stretching exercises, including exercises for mobility and flexibility, are fully discussed starting on page 259. When doing these exercises, start slowly. Gently stretch as far as you can, hold the stretch for 30 seconds, and then ease back. (Studies show that holding a stretch for 30 seconds produces the same result as holding it for 60 seconds). You will feel a gentle stretch but should not have pain or discomfort. As your muscle adapts, the stretch feeling will diminish. You should always perform each exercise slowly and avoid bouncing or forcing the stretch since you could strain a muscle or joint.

Your goal: Try to work up to 20 of each exercise. Do these twice daily in order to maintain a good level of flexibility and strength. As you exercise, remember these tips:

Stretching Tip #1: Always warm your muscles before you start your stretches. Walk or march in place or climb up and down a flight of stairs slowly for a few minutes. Focus on your posture, abdominal control (keeps your spine straight), and regular breathing during this warm-up, which causes circulation of blood to the muscles to increase and helps reduce stiffness and injury. Warm muscles are elastic and will help you to move in full range of motion.

Stretching Tip #2: Listen to your back! Pain is a warning sign. If the stretch or any exercise hurts, stop immediately.

Stretching Tip #3: Remember, the key word is *gentle* stretching. Don't push, bounce, or force the stretch. Although you should feel a stretch, you should never feel pain in the muscle or any other body part. If you do feel pain, stop the stretch immediately.

Stretching Tip #4: Enjoy your stretching time and appreciate how your muscles feel when stretched. This is *not* a competition! Don't try to stretch further than someone else—you may get more than you want in pain or injury.

Strengthening or Resistance Exercises

Strengthening or resistance exercises keep your muscles flexible, strong, and less susceptible to injuries that can cause back pain. When muscles are strong, you are able to perform everyday activities easier, and you will have greater endurance and energy. You can do resistance exercises at a health club, Y, or in the privacy of your own home. As long as the moving muscle has resistance, it will respond. This resistance can come from workout machines, free weights (dumbbells), cans of vegetables from the pantry, elastic bands (available at most sporting goods stores), water (swimming or movement), stairs, a step, an uphill climb, or even your own body weight as you push against a wall or other object.

Resistance exercises support the spine. The soft connective tissues around the spine play a key role in back pain because the large lower back muscles brace the spine. When these muscles become injured or inflamed, they can spasm, resulting in intense pain and limited mobility. Regular strengthening exercises help to keep these large muscles strong and healthy.

When the lower back and abdominal muscles are strong, they stabilize the spine, allow proper spinal movement, and make it easier to maintain correct posture. Strengthening the hip and leg muscles is also important to perform proper lifting techniques and body mechanics, so you can safely lift objects from the floor using your leg muscles rather than reinjure back muscles.

Resistance exercises increase muscle mass. Muscle mass is the metabolically active tissue or tissue that burns calories. The more muscle mass your body has, the more calories you burn each day. Because men have more muscle mass, they burn calories faster and lose weight easier than women. However, with resistance exercises, men and women can increase muscle mass and thus experience weight loss.

If you are still hesitant about staying with a regular resistance exercise program, here's a motivating fact: *Fat burns 2 to 3 calories per pound while muscle burns 50 calories per pound!*

Resistance exercises burn calories. In a study published in November 2002 in the journal *Medicine and Science in Sports and Exercise*, researchers concluded that a person could expend on average 200 to 300 calories during resistance training (size and gender, and the intensity and duration of the workout are factors that affect the average). This is especially good news for those with back pain who want to lose weight while strengthening their back and abdominal muscles. Resistance exercises will let you do both.

Resistance exercises boost optimal health. The American Heart Association reports that regular resistance workouts benefit the cardiovascular system by lowering blood pressure and reducing cholesterol levels, which, in turn, reduce the risk of stroke and heart disease. Resistance exercise is also important in the prevention of sarcopenia, the age-related loss of muscle mass associated with reduced muscle strength and reduced aerobic power.

Resistance exercises help decrease the chance of osteoporosis and bone fractures. Study after study reinforces the positive link between muscle strengthening and osteoporosis prevention in women. In new findings published in the January 2003 issue of *Medicine and Science in Sports and Exercise*, researchers confirmed a significant relationship between total weight lifted by calcium-replete postmenopausal women and a progressive increase in bone density. With more women opting not to use hormone replacement therapy, resistance exercises can fill the gap and help boost bone mass and keep bones strong and fracture free.

Dispelling the Myths

It's important to educate yourself about resistance training. Before we go any further, check out the following myths about resistance exercises—along with some interesting facts:

Myth: *Resistance exercises can increase back pain.*
Truth: If done carefully and with proper technique, resistance exercises can help you build muscle in your abdomen and lower back to keep your posture perfect and support the body's framework. When the spine is supported and flexible, the chance of injury and pain is greatly decreased.

Myth: *If you stop resistance exercises, muscles will turn to fat.*
Truth: This is physiologically impossible. If you stop doing resistance exercises, your muscles will lose size and tone, but it's the excess calories that will be deposited as fat.

Myth: *Resistance exercises can cause even more injury..*

Truth: If done correctly, resistance exercises will help to keep your body fit and strengthen the muscles that support your spine. If you do it improperly, you may get an overuse injury. This happens when people lift weights improperly, lift too much weight, do not rest between exercise sessions, and do not warm up before exercise. The way the muscle builds is by breaking down muscle fibers and allowing the body to regrow these in a stronger way by giving them proper nutrition and rest time. Rest is crucial to gain stronger muscles—and to avoid injury.

Myth: *Resistance exercise means always using heavy equipment.*

Truth: You can easily use the weight of your own body, free weights (hand-held), resistance bands or even the water as resistance.

Myth: *You will get high blood pressure.*

Truth: Resistance exercises do *not* cause high blood pressure. Some people strain their bodies and hold their breath during a lift, which results in a temporary increase of blood pressure. However, this is *never recommended* during resistance exercise.

Myth: *You will become bulky and inflexible.*

Truth: It is important to supplement your resistance exercises with the Pain-Free Back stretching exercises (page 259) to stay flexible.

Pain-Free Back Strengthening Strategies

To start: When doing strengthening exercises, the resistance should be light at first, and then increased gradually as your pain allows and as your strength increases. If you do not have access to light hand or ankle weights or resistance machines, use your hand or a rubber tube or elastic band as resistance.

Start slowly with strengthening exercises, and allow your body time to adjust. If you feel any pain or unusual feeling, stop the exercise. Call your doctor if the pain persists.

When you've mastered the range-of-motion exercises (page 262), add light hand or ankle weights for increased resistance. Starting on page 264, use one- to two-pound weights on the ankles, feet, arms, or hands with the appropriate exercises. Make sure the weights are light (do not exceed two pounds) to avoid adding unnecessary stress to the joints.

Strap the light weights to the hand, wrist, or ankle. If you do not have weights, you can substitute canned goods or pour sand into a thick sock and tie it at the top.

Your goal: I recommend that back pain patients start with 1 or 2 repetitions, twice daily. Gradually increase by 1 or 2 repetitions of each exercise, twice each day, as long as you can do so without pain or fatigue. (Your physical therapist or physician can help you if you have questions about any of the exercises discussed on pages 262–64.) Do the exercises slowly and intentionally, and move your muscles through the full range of motion. The ultimate goal is 20 repetitions of each exercise, twice daily, which may take you months to achieve.

Breathe properly when doing the isometrics or resistance exercises. Never hold your breath during the exercise, and always follow these two steps:

1. Exhale when pushing against the weight or resistance.
2. Inhale when there is little or no resistance.

Allow about two weeks for your muscles to acclimate to the new stresses of resistance exercise. If you stick with your Pain-Free Back strengthening program, you will find that within a few weeks you will start to feel stronger, have better posture, and be able to move around more without stiffness or pain.

Aerobic or Conditioning Exercises

"Why me?" That's one of the first questions patients ask when they are suffering with chronic back pain. Most men and women are greeted with this malady suddenly, such as when they turn to get out of the car, lift groceries out of the trunk, or even roll over in bed during sleep. I explain to all my patients that one of the greatest risk factors for back pain is a sedentary lifestyle. That's why it's important to move around more—all day long.

Aerobic exercise keeps muscles healthy. In addition to the stretching and strengthening (isometric) exercises, I want you to add aerobic or conditioning exercises to your program. An aerobic or conditioning activity is any exercise that increases the heart rate and keeps it higher for a certain period of time. This type of exercise helps your heart and muscles use oxygen more efficiently, and muscles that frequently receive oxygen-rich blood stay healthier. But remember, always start slowly and gradually increase!

Aerobic exercise helps you to maintain a normal weight. Obesity increases the chance of chronic back pain. Losing pounds to get to your normal weight can help end this pain.

Aerobic exercise helps your heart and muscles to work efficiently. By staying active throughout your day, you can go from couch potato to weekday warrior! Aerobic conditioning boosts the amount of oxygen delivered to your heart and muscles, which allows them to work longer. Daily activities such as sweeping a floor, carrying groceries from the car to your home, pushing a lawn mower, or active gardening will improve your aerobic conditioning. Whatever raises your heart rate and keeps it up for a period of time will help you increase endurance.

Water Exercises

For people with a great deal of back pain, water exercises provide a gentle form of conditioning. When other forms of exercise cannot be done because of pain, disability, or decreased bone density, water exercises can give good results since water reduces gravity by 80 percent. The water supports your weight during movement and allows for strengthening and conditioning as you move your body against it.

Stretch in the water, use a kickboard as a floatation device as you push and kick, or swim using slow, gentle strokes. Water exercise can help you to strengthen your muscles and build your cardiovascular endurance.

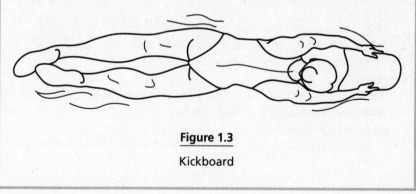

Figure 1.3

Kickboard

Caution: Avoid Overtraining

Overtraining increases the likelihood of fatigue and further back injury. While regular, consistent exercise can help to strengthen the muscles that support your back, excessive exercise (to the point of exhaustion) or overtraining may result in more serious problems.

Pain-Free Back Conditioning Strategies

To start: The following aerobic and conditioning exercises can be helpful for those with back pain:

Biking	Swimming
Gardening	Vacuuming
Hiking	Walking
Housecleaning	Washing windows
Low-impact aerobics	Water exercises
Mall walking	Yard work
Stationary cycling	

Your goal: Do a few minutes of physical activity daily to start, increase by 1 minute or less a session, and work your time up to 60 minutes daily as you gain strength and endurance. Aerobic exercise does not have to take your breath away to be effective. Just move around more—walk,

---

Back Pain Warning Signs

- Severe pain (sharp, shooting, or the electrical shock type) in back
- Pain that is felt in the low back and travels down the back of one leg
- Pain that worsens with movement or activity
- Numbness or tingling
- Inability to extend big toe on the foot that has leg pain
- Weakness of certain leg or foot muscles
- Inability to walk on heel
- Muscle weakness in a leg or foot; bladder or bowel habits are affected.

---

climb stairs, ride a bicycle, dance, walk your dog, or play with kids. Conditioning exercise does not have to be vigorous or continuous. For instance, you can do 5 minutes of movement six times daily or 10 minutes three times daily. Whatever works with your schedule that allows you to move more, do it!

Yoga for Flexibility and Strength

Stress is a leading risk factor for musculoskeletal problems such as back pain. Yoga is an ancient form of exercise that can reduce stress and relieve muscular tension or pain by boosting range of motion and strength. Practicing yoga when you are feeling tense or anxious can help to reduce stress and the risk of injury when you are on the job or at home.

Mark started doing hatha yoga after having surgery to fuse two vertebrae in his lumbar spine following a car accident. After the surgery, this forty-seven-year-old attorney and father of four was told by his surgeon that the back pain might never go away completely and he should "learn to live with it." When Mark could no longer sit in client meetings because of muscle spasms in his back that "took my breath away," he took a leave of absence from his law firm to seek help.

Upon examining Mark, I recommended the *Pain-Free Back Program*. I felt that regular and specific exercise, daily moist heat applications, change in diet to speed up weight loss, and new anti-inflammatory medications would offer him great benefit. I also suggested that he might consider trying hatha yoga, a system made up of breathing practices, meditation, and specific postures that are often beneficial to those with chronic pain. The physical stretching exercises of hatha yoga would help to provide more space for his nerve roots as well as improving flexibility and strengthening Mark's back and abdominal muscles. The breathing techniques would help ease the emotional stress that had built up from living with chronic pain.

Mark started his hatha yoga classes at a studio near his home. Within three weeks, he began to notice a dramatic difference in his pain and stiffness. Because Mark had avoided exercise for almost two years (since the accident), he found it difficult to stretch at first. However, he was determined to get well and soon he was doing gentle stretches and postures along with the more experienced students. After attending class three times a week for three months, Mark experienced dramatic improvement. He could bend more easily, move his arms and neck without fear of

pain, and because his posture was improving and lower back muscles were strengthened, he could even sit for an hour without any discomfort.

Hatha yoga, along with the other steps in the *Pain-Free Back Program*, changed Mark's life. He's now back at work full-time, supporting his family, and continues to attend weekly yoga classes, as well as practicing this discipline at home.

With any type of yoga, you can find great benefits from the physical postures (*asana*) to alleviate aches and pains, concentration exercises (*dharana*) to overcome dwelling on your pain problem, and meditation exercises (*dhyana*) to help you focus on the present instead of ruminating about daily worries.

Physical Postures (Asana) Relieve Pain

The word *asana* means to sit down or sit in a particular position. In yoga, asana refers to the various positions and postures. The asanas are quite useful if your back pain is chronic. The physical postures and daily stretches help to lubricate the body's joints and send nutrients and oxygen to the muscles, bathing them in fresh blood. Taking time to relax and enjoy stretching helps to reduce your blood pressure, relieves stress, and helps you put your pain in perspective.

Concentration Exercises (Dharana) Overcome Worries

The vicious cycle of pain, discussed on page 6, often leads to feelings of depression and worthlessness. Chronic back pain is distressing, but *dharana* or concentration exercises can help to ease the ruminating that robs you of your creativity. The Tree Pose (page 24) helps to calm your anxiety and improve your balance. Other yoga stretches, such as the Child's or Corpse Pose, help you to relax and induce deep sleep.

Meditation (Dhyana) Helps You to Be Mindful

I'll discuss the importance of meditation as a stress and pain reliever in Step 5. For now, know that meditating with yoga—*dhyana*—helps to clear your head and allows you to focus on the "here and now" instead of what might be—or what might have been. Instead of giving in to negative thoughts, you learn to "feel the breath" and calm the mind with yoga poses, which will lead to feelings of inner peace. Yogis feel that people hold emotions deep in the body with the outward signs of hunched shoulders, tight lips, and furrowed brows. Through yoga, we can tap in to these patterns of chronic tightness, release the muscles, and begin to heal the emotional wounds.

Yoga Poses to Try at Home

Child's Pose

This pose can be done several times a day, as needed, to help calm you down. Kneel on the floor on your hands and knees. Your hands should be under the shoulders and your knees under the hips with toes touching. Stretch your neck forward and lengthen your spine through the tailbone. Gently rock the weight of your body back toward your feet, letting your hips stretch farther back as you continue to lengthen and stretch your spine. Stretch your arms forward and walk your fingertips as far forward as they will go on the floor or rug, lengthening your arms fully. Stretch from the shoulders.

As your hips stretch backward, focus on the stretch from the armpits to the hips, lengthening the sides of the torso and the back. If you are flexible, continue stretching and relax your neck as the forehead touches the floor. Pressing the forehead against the floor helps to calm the mind as the forehead and eye muscles completely relax. If this is hard, put one or two pillows under your forehead. Rest a few seconds, allowing the forehead and eye muscles to relax. Let the breath soothe you during this pose. This is a great posture to practice as you prepare for sleep, or if you need a calming moment in a stressful day.

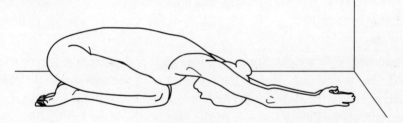

Figure 1.4

The Child's Pose

Tree Pose

This pose is great for improving concentration and practicing meditation, and it also gives the added benefit of building strength and improving balance. Stand with your side next to a wall; use a chair for balance, if you find it difficult to stand on one foot. Stand up straight with big toes touching. Spread the soles of the feet and feel the whole bottom of the feet

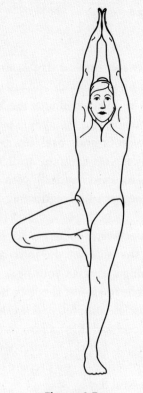

Figure 1.5

The Tree Pose

supporting your weight. Spread the toes wide and engage the leg muscles so the legs feel strong. Rotate the right hip and knee outward so the right knee points to the right wall. The left knee and foot point forward. Lift the right leg and place the sole of the foot on the inner left leg. You can place the foot on the inner ankle, knee, or thigh, depending on your flexibility. Keep the left leg strong and straight, like a tree trunk.

Hold the posture and breathe, keeping the mind calm. If you find it easy to balance on one leg, raise the arms overhead. Continue to keep the left leg strong as you straighten your arms and reach upward toward the sky. Your palms can face each other, or you can bring the palms together. As you reach up, stretch the sides of the torso, keeping the back straight and long. Relax the shoulders and try not to tense the neck and shoulders. Repeat, standing on the right leg, with left leg raised.

Modified Dog Pose

This easy asana helps to build strength and flexibility and can be done anywhere. Stand facing a wall. Spread the soles of the feet and the toes wide for balance. Place the palms of your hands on the wall in front of your waist, and then step back two or three feet, bend forward, and straighten your arms. Press into the wall with your hands, spreading the fingers and palms wide. Engage the hand muscles, wrists, and forearms as you do so. Your back and spine should now be parallel to the floor. Stretch the tailbone away from the wall, and lengthen the sides of the torso from the armpits to the hips. You should feel length through the arms and torso.

Engage the backs of the legs. Now press the heels into the floor and lift the hips toward the ceiling, feeling a nice stretch in the back of the legs. Lift the knee muscles into the quadriceps, and engage the quadriceps as you continue stretching the hamstrings and the back of the legs. Lengthen the arms, torso, and legs as the head and neck relax. Lengthen the neck and release it comfortably. Your body should make a right angle to the wall. This pose is great for relieving back and neck pain.

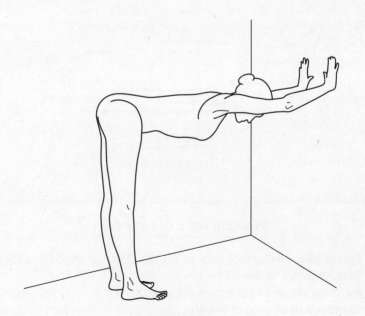

Figure 1.6

The Modified Dog Pose

Corpse Pose

This relaxing pose is a great way to practice meditation. Lie on your back on a comfortable surface, and stretch your arms and legs out straight. Keep your arms down by your sides, and extend your legs straight from the hips. Your feet should be about twelve inches apart, with both feet turned out slightly to keep the feet, ankles, and legs relaxed. With palms facing upward, keep the arms eight to ten inches from the body. Lengthen the back on the floor and feel all muscles stretching and releasing. Notice your shoulder blades and hips, and adjust the body until you feel balanced on both the left and right sides of the body. Scan your body and consciously relax every muscle group, including the throat, face, and eye muscles. Continue this scanning as you lie down and relax, and become aware of areas in which you might hold chronic tension.

As you lie there, feel the breath take you into a deeper relaxed state. The more you practice meditation in this pose, the easier it will become to still the thoughts. As you practice meditation, do not criticize yourself if you cannot quiet your mind, just accept yourself as you are. With time, the practice of meditation becomes more calming and you will feel more rejuvenated.

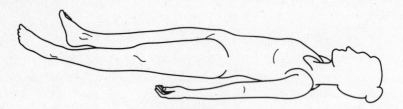

Figure 1.7

The Corpse Pose

Warning Signs of Neck Pain

- Severe pain (sharp, shooting, or like an electrical shock) in back of neck, shoulder, or down one arm
- Pain that worsens with movement or activity
- Numbness or tingling in one arm
- Weakness of arm muscles

Neck Pain—When to Call the Doctor

- Mild neck pain that persists for 3 or 4 days after self-treatment
- Severe neck pain or arm pain
- Neck pain or neck and arm pain that goes away for short periods but keeps coming back
- New or unexplained symptoms appear

Tai Chi Helps Increase Mobility

There are several excellent studies on tai chi helping older men and women increase mobility and body mechanics. The series of flowing, graceful movements with tai chi not only give participants a good workout and stretching regimen, but also increase their sense of balance, ability to bend, and capacity to do household tasks. Because older adults are at increased risk of falling, tai chi can help them avoid falling and injury, as well as keep their backs flexible and strong. Talk to your doctor or contact a local studio for personal instruction.

Exercise Blunders That Can Increase Pain

Avoid the following exercises at first since they might aggravate back or neck pain:

1. Leg lifts, lifting both legs together while lying on your back
2. Sit-ups keeping both legs straight
3. Sit-ups with bent legs
4. Lifting heavy hand weights above the waist
5. Stretching while sitting with the legs in a V position
6. Toes touching while standing with both legs straight
7. Twisting or turning your neck in "circles"
8. Bending the neck forward or looking up

Pain-Free Back Rx

Now that you know why you must exercise to get well, are you ready to get started? Here's the first thing to do: read the chart on page xv to make sure you don't have a more serious form of back pain, such as a compression fracture or kidney stone. If any of the descriptions in the chart apply to your situation, see your doctor before starting this exercise program.

Now, when you can sit comfortably, you can begin exercising. For the first few days, I recommend starting exercise by walking around your home until you can do it without pain. You may only be able to do this for less than a minute the first time—and that's perfectly fine. Just increase the time you walk, starting with a minute or less, and gradually increase by a minute a day if you can.

Follow this Pain-Free Back rule: When you finish walking (or exercising), you should have no more pain than when you started. If your pain is dramatically worse, check with your doctor. You could have a more serious problem that needs medical attention.

Avoid activities that involve twisting, bending, or high impact, or that make your back hurt more. If you have a tendency to get attacks of low back pain, you should continue the exercises indefinitely to prevent new attacks.

Walk, Don't Run!

You don't have to run a marathon to get fit and alleviate your back pain. In fact, that would probably be the worst thing you could do, as high-intensity exercise would stress you physically and set you up for injury. *Remember, you only get one back for life—protect it!*

Review the Pain-Free Back exercises. Before you start your Pain-Free Back Exercise Program, choose low-impact activities that you enjoy (see list on page 29) and that you will regularly do. Review the exercises on page 259. Make sure you understand how these exercises are performed, and if you have questions, talk to your doctor or a physical therapist for instructions.

Block 35 minutes each day for exercise. After you are able to move easier, allow 35 minutes to do your entire daily exercise regimen. Block this time on your calendar each day so you know you will make the commitment, and don't let anyone or anything stop your Pain-Free Back Exercise Program. Would you let them stop you from taking prescribed medication? This program is your *free ticket* for a pain-free back and increased mobility. As you feel stronger and have less pain, extend this exercise time, adding more stretches and exercising more throughout your day.

Alternate your exercise regimen. For four days each week, you will focus on stretching and aerobic exercise. On the alternating three days, you will focus on stretching and resistance exercise. Be sure to allow one day of rest after resistance exercise so the muscle can respond to the workout. When you are able to exercise, here is the schedule to follow:

4 Days Each Week

Time	Type of Exercise or Activity
5 minutes	Warm-up (walk in place or do any light exercise)
10 minutes	Stretches (see page 14)
15 minutes	Aerobic activity (walking, biking, swimming)
5 minutes	Cooldown (walk in place or do any light exercise again)

3 Days Each Week (Alternate Days)

Time	Type of Exercise or Activity
5 minutes	Warm-up (walk in place or do any light exercise)
10 minutes	Stretches (see page 14)
15 minutes	Strengthening exercises (follow page 15)
5 minutes	Cooldown (walk in place or do any light exercise again)

Exercise with a Friend

Almost all of my patients who tell of exercising with their spouse or a friend have greater success with the Pain-Free Back Exercise Program than those who try to do it alone. The exercise partner can act as a coach, motivator, and conscience—as well as someone to talk to during exercise. In an interesting study from Indiana University's Department of Kinesiology, researchers found that spouses who worked out with their partners had a dropout rate of only 6.3 percent compared with spouses who worked out without their partners. The "single" exercising group had an astounding 43 percent dropout rate.

Join an Exercise Group

You might also consider joining a fitness classes at a local health club, Y, or school. Or check out the mall—most enclosed shopping centers sponsor early morning mall walking groups. Some even have medical personnel who monitor blood pressure, do regular health screenings, or answer health questions.

Build Your Own Home Gym

If you'd rather exercise in the comfort of your own home, you're not alone. Many people enjoy exercising in private. Exercising at home allows you to choose the time of day and exercise at your own pace. In addition, with all the new home exercise equipment and videotapes, all you have to do is pop in the tape or use the machine to get moving—no matter how inclement the weather is outside.

If you are just getting started with exercise, read the classified advertisements for used exercise equipment such as electronic treadmills or stationary bicycles. Online auctions usually have these for sale and at greatly reduced prices. Some basics you might consider include

- Rubber mats for doing stretches and yoga postures
- Light weights
- Workout gloves to protect your hands from holding the weights
- Exercise bands or tubes
- Instructional videos for beginning yoga, tai chi, and stretching exercises
- A "fit ball," which are used by physical therapists for stretching the lower back and doing abdominal work (be sure to ask your physical therapist for proper instructions)
- A full-length mirror to make sure your posture is correct during your stretching and other exercises

Hire a Personal Trainer to Get Started

Get a personal trainer to help you keep track of your progress, give you lots of encouragement, and schedule your workouts for you. Call your local Y for referrals or check in the Yellow Pages. You'll need to interview several to find the right person, and consider paying for three months to get into the exercise habit to end back pain. Make sure your trainer has at least a bachelor's degree in exercise science or a related health-science discipline, experience, and certification from an internationally recognized organization like the American College of Sports Medicine, the American Council on Exercise, or the National Strength and Conditioning Association. You'll be surprised at how much progress you'll make with a trainer who will make sure you stick with your required regimen.

Consider Physical Therapy

Consider consulting with a physical therapist or an American College of Sports Medicine certified exercise specialist, if needed, to find which exercises are best for your body and your specific type of back pain. It's better to know proper form ahead of time than deal with aches and pains from yet another injury. Physical therapy can be prescribed by your doctor and is generally covered by insurance. Generally, physical therapists and physicians work together to provide you with the best care.

3 Pain-Relieving Back Savers

Use Moist Heat before and after Exercise

Using moist heat applications on your back or painful area before and after exercise may help you to stay with your program until your muscles strengthen and the pain subsides. Heat increases blood flow to the site and decreases joint stiffness. Regular moist heat applications also alleviate pain temporarily, reduce muscle spasms, and help to decrease inflammation.

When using moist heat, make sure it is not too warm, or else you can burn your skin. Use the moist heat application for at least 15 minutes before exercise, and then use it again immediately following exercise. (You can also use moist heat any time you want additional relief from back pain.) Some patients find great relief by doing their exercises in a hot tub or sitting on a stool (with rubber tips for safety) under a warm shower (comfortable but not too hot). The constant heat flowing on the affected site helps to keep pain minimal and allows for easier movement. Choose from the following popular types of moist heat:

- Warm shower (sit on chair, if needed)
- Warm, moist towel or cloth
- Warm bath
- Warm whirlpool or hot tub

Heat Wrap Therapy

A new heat therapy is giving good results for patients with back pain. A study in the journal *Spine* reported that heat may be a better alternative for relieving lower back pain than the over-the-counter medications ibuprofen (Advil, Motrin, and others) and acetaminophen (Tylenol and others). The study of 371 people with lower back pain found that a 40-degree Celsius (104° F) heat wrap worn for eight hours a day improved muscle stiffness and flexibility more than either drug.

The heat is delivered continuously at the site of pain for eight hours. You can safely use this form of heat therapy during the day or night, even while sleeping, for optimal pain relief. This disposable heat patch or belt can be purchased at your local pharmacy or at online drugstores.

- Heated swimming pool
- Hot packs (some can be warmed in a microwave, such as the Bed Buddy brand)
- Moist heating pad
- Paraffin–mineral oil therapeutic mixture

Backsaver #2: Try Cold Therapy

If heat doesn't work, try cold therapy. Use ice or cold packs, though do not *ever* apply the ice directly to your skin or you might experience more than back pain! You might also try a local spray such as fluromethane (nonflammable) on your back or painful area before and after exercise. This superficial cooling decreases muscle spasms and raises the threshold of pain. Some patients prefer cold therapy to moist heat for acute back pain, while others tell of getting the best relief by alternating the sessions of moist heat and ice. I suggest that you choose the method of moist heat and ice packs that gives the *best relief with the least trouble or expense.* (Always use caution to avoid damage to your skin with hot and cold therapies.)

Backsaver #3: Take Medications

Although you should not rely on medications to "cure" your back pain, they are an integral part of a comprehensive treatment plan to reduce inflammation and pain and stop muscle spasm. Some medications will

USE R.I.C.E. for Injuries

If your pain stems from a muscle injury, treat it immediately with RICE: Rest, Ice, Compression, and Elevation. Rest the injured body part, and then apply ice (an ice pack or bag of frozen vegetables or fruit) for 20 minutes on, then 20 minutes off. Add compression with a firm elastic bandage. Elevate the injured part to keep swelling minimal. If the muscles of the back are the problem, lie on your back and prop your legs on top of a chair or bench (see page 111 for position) to relieve pressure on the back.

help to control severe pain, which will let you start exercising sooner. The faster you begin to move and strengthen your muscles, the greater long-term improvement you'll see.

In the severe acute phase of back pain, some medications (analgesics) are used purely for pain control, when needed. Other medications help pain and inflammation (anti-inflammatory drugs), and still others help muscle tightness and spasms (muscle relaxants). For chronic pain, meaning pain that has lasted longer than expected or for more than three months, other medications are used to allow you to have pain control and be active. All of the recommended Pain-Free Back medications are discussed fully on pages 186–200.

Sample Weekly Chart for the Pain-Free Back Exercise Program

Day of Week	Type of Exercise	Time (in Minutes)	Moist Heat or Ice	Medication
Monday	Warm-up	5	Moist heat/ shower before and after	Advil (ibuprofen)
	Stretches	10		
	Walk on treadmill	15		
	Cooldown	5		
Tuesday	Warm-up	5	Moist heat followed by ice packs after exercise	Advil (ibuprofen)
	Stretches	10		
	Resistance exercises	15		
	Cooldown	5		

Sample Weekly Chart *(continued)*

Day of Week	Type of Exercise	Time (in Minutes)	Moist Heat or Ice	Medication
Wednesday	Warm-up	5	Hot tub before	Advil
	Stretches	10	and after	(ibuprofen)
	Swim in pool	15	exercise;	
	Cooldown	5	ice pack before	
			bedtime	
Thursday	Warm-up	5	Warm shower	Tylenol
	Stretches	10	followed by ice	(acetamino-
	Resistance		packs; hot tub	phen)
	exercises	15	before bedtime	
	Cooldown	5		
Friday	Warm-up	5	Hot tub before	Advil
	Stretches	10	and after	(ibuprofen)
	Stationary bike	15	exercise; warm	
	Cooldown	5	shower before	
			bedtime	
Saturday	Warm-up	5	Ice therapy	Advil
	Stretches	10	before and	(ibuprofen)
	Resistance		after exercise;	
	exercises	15	moist heating	
	Cooldown	5	pad on back	
			before bedtime	
Sunday	Warm-up	5	Hot tub before	Advil
	Stretches	10	and after	(ibuprofen)
	Swim in pool	15	exercise; heat-	
	Cooldown	5	wrap therapy	
			all night during	
			sleep	

The Pain-Free Back
Healthy Eating Plan

At her heaviest, Kelly weighed in at 205 pounds. This thirty-nine-year-old woman had maintained a normal weight for most of her life. When she was pregnant with twins, however, she gained more than 85 pounds. Because of complications four months into the pregnancy, Kelly's doctor prescribed bed rest until delivery. Once the twins were born, Kelly realized what constant bed rest and lack of exercise could do to a person—she was obese and had no energy or muscle tone. Even picking up her newborns was difficult because her arms were so weak. Then one day, while pushing the twins' double-stroller on a morning outing, Kelly turned to wave to a friend and felt a "pop" in her back.

"My lower back went out completely," she said. "I could not even turn around to push the stroller. With each movement or turn, the pain was excruciating and brought tears to my eyes. Luckily, my friend came and helped me get the twins back home. I called my husband, and I went to bed."

Kelly stayed in bed for several days, thinking that this would put an end to the tremendous pain and stiffness she felt. When the pain and other symptoms worsened, she came to see me for an evaluation.

Although Kelly could take medication to ease her pain, it's difficult to find easy answers for a case like hers, since many risk factors greatly increased her chances of pain or back injury. Not only was she seriously overweight, but Kelly also had very poor muscle tone, was unfit, and was recovering from a difficult labor and childbirth.

After doing an examination, I told Kelly that it was most likely that the pain was from muscles and tendons in the back—soft tissue pain. I felt it was important that she work on losing the excess weight and explained to her that being overweight by more than 20 pounds greatly increases the risk of back pain. Because Kelly had gained so much weight and had been sedentary for so long, she felt tired and uncomfortable exercising. Weight loss would be a great start to help her enjoy moving around more, and the increased activity would result in further weight loss and resolve her pain.

Kelly started the Pain-Free Back Healthy Eating Plan, watching her portion sizes, focusing on a diet higher in protein and lower in carbohydrates, and eating five smaller meals per day instead of three large meals. The carefully selected mini-meals helped Kelly avoid snacking out of boredom, which had been her habit for months. Eating frequently also gave her a boost in energy so she could take her twins on regular strolls through her neighborhood.

Kelly was not breast-feeding her twins, so I prescribed a nonsteroidal anti-inflammatory medication (NSAID), which allowed her to move more without pain and start a stretching program. I also recommended that she use moist heat applications twice daily, or more often if they gave relief for her pain and stiffness. Kelly said she studied yoga in college, so she agreed to do yoga positions at home.

This young mother realized that to have the strength to care for her new infants, she had to take serious measures to lose the extra weight and get fit again—and she did just that. Her first step was cleaning out the kitchen cupboards, which were filled with junk foods, processed or prepared foods, and colas. (Kelly admitted that she had lived on junk food and quick and easy meals while lying in bed for five months.) Kelly then went to the local farmer's market and stocked up on fresh produce—fruits and vegetables, as well as whole grains, soy products, fresh fish, and lentils. When she went grocery shopping, she shopped the perimeter of the store where the fresh produce and meats were kept and avoided the middle aisles where the packaged foods were sold.

Just as she promised, Kelly stayed with the Pain-Free Back Healthy Eating Plan and started regular stretching exercises, taking it very slowly at first because of the pain. She did the moist heat applications and found that a warm bubble bath in the evening helped her relax from her busy day as a new mom and also alleviated pain and stiffness. Within two weeks after her injury, Kelly started yoga, doing a few poses at first and slowly building to doing these several times each day, as she felt stronger and less pain.

When Kelly came back to see me five months later, she was like a new

---

Use Your Pain-Free Back Diary

As you start Your Pain-Free Back Healthy Eating Plan, use the diary (or PDA), suggested on page 4, to keep a detailed record of what you eat each day. By writing down everything you eat, along with the serving size, it will help increase your awareness of why you might be overweight. For instance, you may think you are eating a healthful diet, watching your portions, then after calculating your calories or carbohydrates at the end of the day, find you have eaten twice as many as you thought (not uncommon!).

Interestingly, studies have shown that when researchers ask obese people to record their daily food intake, the results are surprising. The same people who said they ate no more than 1,100 calories per day topped off at an average of over 2,000 calories per day. When researchers told people their actual caloric intake, they became more aware of portion sizes and calorie counts.

Use your Pain-Free Back Diary just as you would a checkbook, writing down what you eat each day, the portion size, and calorie or carbohydrate counts, depending on the weight-loss program you undertake. As you go through the day, add up the calories or carbohydrates in your diet. If you are over the suggested limits, make adjustments the next day.

If you find you still cannot get in control of your weight, talk to a registered dietitian for a personalized weight-loss program.

---

person. She had dropped fifty pounds and looked ten years younger from the weight loss and exercise. Kelly said her energy level was tremendous. Her pain had completely resolved, and she continued to do her daily yoga postures, twice-daily stretches, and regular aerobic walking while pushing the twins in their stroller. Kelly now knows what it takes to keep her back strong and has vowed to stay at this normal weight forever.

Banish Back Pain with Weight Loss

Next to exercising daily, the most important thing you can do to end back pain is to lose weight or maintain an ideal weight. It is estimated that in the United States, approximately 61 percent (110 million) of adults (aged twenty to seventy-four) are overweight or obese. The Centers for Disease

Control and Prevention (CDC) has indicated that the rate of obesity has increased in all fifty states in 2002. Moreover, childhood obesity has reached its highest level in thirty years. Contributing to these figures is the fact that Americans are exercising less and eating more calories than ever before.

What Is Your Ideal Body Weight?
Most people have no idea what their ideal weight might be. I tell my patients that a healthy weight is one at which you are comfortable, do not have weight-related diseases (such as high blood pressure, heart disease, and diabetes), and are not likely to develop those diseases in the future. Some new research shows that Body Mass Index (BMI) may be the best indicator of a healthy—or unhealthy—weight. Your BMI represents the relationship between weight and height and correlates with body fat.

For adults aged twenty years or older, the BMI falls into one of four categories: underweight, normal, overweight, or obese. At this time, it is estimated that about 64.5 percent of adults are overweight with a body mass index of 25+, and more than 30 percent of those are obese with a BMI of 30+. These statistics are startling to me. Of course, some people who have an "overweight" BMI may have a normal amount of body fat with a large muscle mass, and others who have a "normal" BMI may have excess fat and reduced muscle mass. However, on average, these statistics hold true and are a warning sign to all Americans who consume more food than necessary.

Determine your BMI: Using your height and weight, find your BMI number as established by the National Institutes of Health (figure 2.1):

Category	BMI
Underweight	18.5 or less
Normal weight	18.5–24.9
Overweight	25–29.9
Obese	30 or more

What the BMI number means: Obesity or a high BMI is associated with chronic illness such as heart disease, diabetes, and arthritis. It makes good sense that getting to an ideal weight (BMI of 18.5 to 24.9) will help reduce the risk of chronic illness, resolve your back pain, and return you to an active life again.

	120	130	140	150	160	170	180	190	200	210	220	230	240	250	260	270	280	290	300	310	320	330
4'5"	30	33	35	38	40	43	45	48	50	53	55	58	60	63	65	68	70	73	75	78	80	83
4'6"	29	31	34	36	39	41	43	46	48	51	53	55	58	60	63	65	67	70	72	75	77	80
4'7"	29	30	33	35	37	40	42	44	46	49	51	53	56	58	60	63	65	67	70	72	74	77
4'8"	27	29	31	34	36	38	40	43	45	47	49	52	54	56	58	61	63	65	67	69	72	74
4'9"	26	28	30	32	35	37	39	41	44	46	48	50	52	54	56	58	61	63	65	67	69	71
4'10"	25	27	29	31	33	36	38	40	42	44	46	48	50	52	54	56	59	61	63	65	67	69
4'11"	24	26	28	30	32	35	36	38	41	43	45	47	49	51	53	55	57	59	61	63	65	67
5'0"	23	25	27	29	31	33	35	37	40	41	43	45	47	49	51	53	55	57	59	61	63	64
5'1"	23	25	26	28	30	32	34	36	38	40	42	43	45	47	49	51	53	55	57	59	60	62
5'2"	22	24	26	27	29	31	33	35	37	38	40	42	44	46	48	50	51	53	55	57	59	60
5'3"	21	23	25	27	28	30	32	34	35	37	39	41	43	44	46	48	50	51	53	55	57	59
5'4"	21	22	24	26	27	29	31	32	34	36	38	39	41	43	45	46	48	50	51	53	55	57
5'5"	20	22	23	25	27	28	30	32	33	35	37	38	40	42	43	45	47	48	50	52	53	55
5'6"	19	21	23	24	26	27	29	31	32	34	36	37	39	40	42	44	45	47	48	50	52	53
5'7"	19	20	22	23	25	27	28	30	31	33	34	36	38	39	41	42	44	46	47	49	50	52
5'8"	18	20	21	23	24	26	27	29	30	32	33	35	36	38	40	41	43	44	46	47	49	50
5'9"	18	19	21	22	24	25	27	28	30	31	33	34	35	37	38	40	41	43	44	46	47	49
5'10"	17	19	20	22	23	24	26	27	29	30	32	33	34	36	37	39	40	42	43	44	46	47
5'11"	17	18	20	21	23	24	25	26	28	29	31	32	33	35	36	37	39	40	42	43	45	46
6'0"	16	18	19	20	22	23	24	26	27	28	30	31	33	34	35	37	38	39	41	42	43	45
6'1"	16	17	18	20	21	22	24	25	26	28	29	30	32	33	34	36	37	39	40	41	42	44
6'2"	15	17	18	19	21	22	23	24	26	27	28	30	31	33	34	35	36	37	39	40	41	42
6'3"	15	16	17	19	20	21	22	24	25	26	27	29	30	31	32	34	35	36	37	39	40	41
6'4"	15	16	17	18	19	21	22	23	24	26	27	28	29	30	32	33	34	35	37	38	39	40
6'5"	14	15	17	18	19	20	21	23	24	25	26	27	28	30	31	32	33	34	36	37	38	39
6'6"	14	15	16	17	18	20	21	22	23	24	25	27	28	29	30	31	32	34	35	36	37	38
6'7"	14	15	16	17	18	19	20	21	23	24	25	26	27	28	29	30	32	33	34	35	36	37
6'8"	13	14	15	16	18	19	20	21	22	23	24	25	26	27	29	30	31	32	33	34	35	36
6'9"	13	14	15	16	17	18	19	20	21	23	24	25	26	27	28	29	30	31	32	33	34	35
6'10"	13	14	15	16	17	18	19	20	21	22	23	24	25	26	27	28	29	30	31	32	33	35

Figure 2.1

Body Mass Index Chart

Speaking of Calories . . .

Although we used to believe that counting fat grams would allow you to lose weight, we now know this is not always the case. It is true that fat is calorie dense, with nine calories per gram, and that limiting foods loaded with fat automatically limits your calorie intake, leading to weight loss. Carbohydrates and protein, on the other hand, provide less than half the calories of fat or about four calories per gram.

Now, new studies on very-low-carbohydrate diets (defined as less than 50 grams of carbohydrate per day) have given us confusing results. Most studies report that people lose more weight on a very-low-carbohydrate diet than on a diet that contains the same amount of calories but more carbohydrates. While some of this additional weight loss might be attributed to water loss, researchers believe that these diets alter the metabolic rate of the body. Assessments of body composition with very-low-carbohydrate diets indicate a greater loss of fat mass while the lean body mass is preserved. This suggests that the very-low-carbohydrate diet favors loss of fat. That's good news!

Nonetheless, eating as much as you want of any food is certainly not the answer to weight loss. Until we know differently, keep a tally of your daily calories to know what's going into your body. We still believe that if you eat more calories than you burn off, you will gain weight.

As a physician, I still believe that calories are important. Whether you stay on a low-carb, high-protein diet or prefer the more traditional low-fat diet, it's important to burn more calories than you take in to lose weight.

For weight loss, take the weight you want to be (make this a reasonable weight for your height), add a zero to that number and eat no fewer than that number of calories per day. This may seem simplistic, but it does prevent people from eating a calorie level below their basal metabolic rate and possibly affecting their metabolism. More important, restricting your calories too much could cause you to binge, as you will not be able to maintain this behavior for a long period of time.

Personal Calorie Target

Ideal Body Weight X 10 = Minimum Calories Per Day

Check Your Waist-to-Hip Ratio

For back pain sufferers, the one problem you need to watch out for is a large abdomen. Not only is an expanding waistline uncomfortable, making it difficult to move and breathe, but a large stomach can greatly increase your back pain. In addition, men who have a waist size larger than 40 inches have three times the risk for diabetes, high blood pressure, and high cholesterol than men with smaller waist sizes. High cholesterol leads to heart disease, heart attack, and heart failure. Women who have large waists or apple shapes are more likely to have persistent activation of blood cells called platelets, which leads to increased blood clotting and may boost heart attack and stroke risk.

In a large Japanese study published in 2000 in the *Archives of Internal Medicine*, researchers found that the waist-to-hip ratio was higher in women with generalized back pain, meaning that these women were more likely than others to have excess abdominal fat. They also, on average, had less muscle in their back and legs than other study participants. Another study, published in 1997 in the *International Journal of Obesity and Related Metabolic Disorders*, concluded that women with large waists have a significantly increased likelihood of low back pain. A study published in 1998 in the *American Journal of Public Health* reached the same conclusion: large waist circumferences and high BMIs are more likely to be associated with impaired quality of life and disability affecting basic activities of daily living. A large abdomen can cause postural changes resulting in prolonged overstretching of ligaments and other soft tissues, and increased compression on joints and disks. Your back will try to support the extra weight in front by swaying backwards, causing excess strain on the lower back muscles. Excess weight and muscle imbalance increase stress on joints and soft tissues.

Apple or pear?
Some scientists put us in various categories, depending on the way we are built. For example, there are those men and women we call "apples," who accumulate fat at the waistline (mostly men). Pears (mostly women) are those that carry more weight below the waist and around the thighs and upper legs. If you are an apple body type, you have a higher risk of developing heart disease, diabetes, high blood pressure, stroke, and even some cancers—and you have an increased risk of suffering with back pain.

Determine your shape.
Here's a simple formula to tell if you are an apple or pear: Break out your measuring tape, measure your waist in inches at its narrowest point, and then divide that figure by your hip measurement at the widest point. For

women the apple/pear score should not exceed *0.80*. For men the score should not exceed *0.95*.

For instance, Denise, a pear, has a waist measurement of 31 inches and a hip measurement of 42.

31 divided by 42 = .73 (**acceptable**—less than .80)

Ginah's figure is definitely an apple since her waist is 38 and her hips are 40.

38 divided by 40 = .96 (**too high**—greater than .80)

Raymond is an apple as well, with a waist at 38 and hips at 38.

38 divided by 38 = 1 (**too high**—greater than men's .95)

Personal Waist/Hip Score

Waist (in inches _____ ÷ Hip (in inches) ____ = _____

Whether you are an apple or a pear with a growing waistline, it's time to do something positive for your body and your back as you start to lose that visceral body fat, the type that hides deep within the recesses of the body, close to organs and increases your risk of heart disease and diabetes.

Now Take Action

Most adults know how to lose weight if they are overweight. After all, with the use of the Internet, you can go on any popular health website and download meal plans to boost weight loss, depending on the foods you enjoy eating. On the other hand, your doctor can give you a standard "office diet" that is reasonable for weight loss.

Over the past twenty-five years in consulting with thousands of back pain patients on losing weight, I've concluded there are several recommendations that remain "tried and true," no matter what the latest fads are, and I will give you these weight loss tips in this step. These suggestions will help you to lose weight slowly and keep the weight off for good, if you stick with the Pain-Free Back Healthy Eating Plan. The tips are not difficult, and allow you to eat more food than you normally would on a very low fat diet.

Stop Drinking Soda

If you eliminate one cola a day (about 150 calories), this adds up to more than 50,000 calories annually or a weight reduction of 15 pounds.

The Pain-Free Back Diet

Without knowing your medical history or consulting with you in person, it is difficult to prescribe a personalized weight loss plan that will meet your health needs. After all, what works for one person may be very wrong for someone else. What I will do in Step 2 is present you with suggestions that have worked with thousands of my patients. These tips will give you an overview of how to jump-start your weight loss, so you can feel good about your efforts and see results. Once you lose 5 to 10 pounds, begin to add more food choices with your specific health and dietary needs in mind.

I do know that if you follow the Pain-Free Back Healthy Eating Plan, you will lose weight. I've seen it work again and again as men and women get a quick start on weight loss, see good results, and then slowly take weight off without feeling hungry or fatigued.

Pain-Free Back Weight-Loss Tip #1:
Jump-Start Weight Loss with a
High-Protein, Low-Carbohydrate Diet
Low-carbohydrate (low-carb) diets are the rage now among consumers, and with reason. They are also becoming more accepted by the medical community. You can read about them on the Internet, and the media releases news almost daily on new low-carb findings. Also, a host of new low-carb, high-protein bars, shakes, and other foods are available that are quite tasty.

Always curious about finding results-oriented diets for my patients, I've spent a lot of time researching the myriad low-carb diets out there. I've also assessed my patients who successfully followed low-carb diets and have found these diets can truly *jump-start weight loss*. Not only do you block hunger with the low-carb/high-protein/fat combination, but you'll also see *fast results*. For most people, results are a superb motivating tool to help them stick with a diet and get to an ideal weight. I believe patient compliance is greater with the low-carb, high-protein diet, and if you carefully make healthy choices, you will feel great while dropping pounds.

Controlled carbohydrate weight-loss diets usually contain no more than 25 percent of the energy as carbohydrates, although some may have more or less. The one thing they all have in common is that they suppress appetite and increase the metabolic rate—key factors in permanent weight loss.

In the past year, more studies are coming out confirming that a low-carb, high-protein diet may be just what the doctor ordered for some people. For example, in the November 2002 issue of the *Cleveland Clinic Journal of Medicine*, researchers examined approximately fifty scientific studies featuring very-low-carbohydrate diets (less than 50 grams of carbohydrate per day). Based on the hypothesis, the scientists concluded that there was a lack of scientific evidence for the criticisms against low-carb diets. Indeed, some of their findings revealed a significant amount of data showing positive metabolic responses to very-low-carbohydrate diets.

In the Cleveland Clinic findings, researchers presented the following key points:

- Much of the criticism of low-carb diets is based on a misunderstanding of what a low-carb diet entails.
- Comparing low-carb diets to standard weight-loss diets, people lose more weight on very-low-carbohydrate diets than on standard weight-loss diets.
- Mechanisms of weight loss on very-low-carbohydrate diets may go beyond water loss, and include appetite suppression and increasing the metabolic rate.
- Weight loss is usually associated with reductions in lean body mass, but individuals following a very-low-carbohydrate diet tend to lose less lean body mass compared with individuals following a low-fat diet.
- Very-low-carbohydrate diets have favorable effects on cardiovascular disease risk factors.

I believe that the next five years will be fairly significant as more scientific findings conclude that there are ways to lose weight that differ from the standard "low-calorie" or "low-fat" diets. I also know that because people are all different, we have to try different eating plans to find the *right one* that suits our personal tastes and needs—and gives us results.

Several high-protein diets are currently touted in the marketplace, including the popular high-protein, low-carb diet developed by Dr. Atkins; the one in the book, *The Zone*, by Dr. Barry Sears; and Sugar Busters, by a group of physicians. Though each diet has enthusiastic fans and critics, you simply have to do your own homework and then talk with your doctor about the one that works best for your health and your weight-loss goals.

For example, I have patients who are vegetarians, and together we have found that a modified version of the high-protein, low-carb diet works in weight loss and minimizing hunger. These men and women eat an array of soy products, veggie burgers, fresh fruits and vegetables, seeds and nuts, and low-fat dairy products, among other foods. They still keep a count on their carbs each day and have reported incredible results. Other patients have told of doing a modified lower saturated fat, low-carb diet using skinless chicken, fish, lean beef, low-fat cheese, vegetables, fruits, and soy products. They, too, stay within a certain carbohydrate daily limit, and all of these patients have lost weight. There are also new products such as Nature's Own™ low-carbohydrate bread that can be used effectively on a low-carb eating plan.

I believe there is not just one "set in stone" rule of what you can or cannot eat to lose weight and be healthy. Successful weight loss using any dietary plan means finding healthful foods that work to keep you well and at an ideal weight and then integrating these foods into your daily meal plan. (See the Pain-Free Back Recipes starting on page 215.)

The Atkins Diet
While most people think of the Atkins diet as eating just meat, it isn't at all about eating meat, but rather about cutting back on refined carbohydrates, including white bread, pasta, rice, crackers, snacks, sugary desserts, and more. This nutritional approach to weight loss is designed to prevent blood sugar levels from spiking and causing the overproduction

---

Caution

Before starting any new diet, talk to your doctor to make sure it is appropriate. If you have kidney disease, diabetes, heart disease, or any other chronic health problem, it's imperative that you discuss any new eating plan with your doctor or with a registered dietitian.

of insulin—a hormone that helps convert carbohydrates to body fat. One patient who followed this diet and lost more than sixty pounds said, "I eat fresh whole vegetables, fruits, lean meat, soy products, cheese, and fish instead of potato chips, french fries, chocolate shakes, and cookies. I think the low-carb way to eat is much healthier than stuffing on snacks and fast food all day."

On the Atkins diet, some studies show that people can lose twice as much weight as on the standard low-fat, high-carbohydrate approach. In addition, though there has been great negative debate about this diet, some newer medical studies provide reports that this diet does *not* drive up the risk of heart disease—that cholesterol, triglycerides, and blood pressure often improve. As a physician, I realize this improvement could be related to the weight loss itself, but if that's the case, I'm glad the patient dropped the weight.

Perhaps one of the reasons why patients are compliant with staying on the diet is that the combination of fat and protein satisfy the appetite, so you are simply not hungry. Stable blood sugar throughout the day ensures that you will have fewer food cravings and fewer false hunger pains. Alternately, eating lots of carbohydrates as with the standard high-carb, low-fat diet sends insulin levels soaring, lowers blood sugar, and eventually makes you famished. Of course, not everyone reacts to carbohydrates in this manner, but if you do get hungry after a high-carb meal, such as a plate of pasta with red sauce, a baked potato topped with sour cream and chives, or large bagel with "lite" cream cheese, the Atkins diet may help to curb your hunger pangs.

Studies are coming in showing that you can eat more on the Atkins diet and still lose weight. For instance, in a study from Mount Sinai Medical Center in New York City, researchers put overweight teenagers on comparison diets for two months. The teens on the Atkins diet lost twice as much as those on the low-fat diet, yet the "Atkins teens" ate about 700 more calories a day than the others. In another comprehensive study from the University of Cincinnati, women who followed the Atkins plan lost twice as much while eating the same number of calories as the low-fat dieters.

A most revealing study published in the February 2003 issue of the *Journal of Nutrition* came to the same conclusion, that the high-protein diet gives a weight-loss advantage. In this study, researchers from the University of Illinois studied the amino acid leucine (in high-protein animal foods such as beef, chicken, fish) and found that it plays a major role in losing fat and maintaining muscle. In the study twenty-four middle-aged women with an average weight of 182 pounds consumed about 1,700 calories per day. The protein-rich group took in about 30 percent of their calories from protein, 41 percent from carbohydrates, and 29 percent from fat. The women ate about 10 ounces of meat every day over the ten-week study—including one beef serving—as well as three servings of low-fat milk or cheese and at least five servings of vegetables. Meanwhile, the high-carbohydrate group ate only half as much protein, getting 16 percent of their total calories in protein, 58 percent from carbohydrates, and 26 percent from fat.

The women averaged about 16 pounds in weight loss, but those who followed the low-carb, high-protein plan reportedly lost more body fat and retained more lean muscle than the women who followed the high-carbohydrate dietary plan. Several months after the study was concluded, researchers found that the high-protein group continued to lose weight while the high-carbohydrate group did not.

Realizing that about 95 percent of people who go on weight-loss diets will gain all or some of it back within a year, the very thing to consider if you have tried to lose weight without success might be a new eating style. Moreover, I might add, weight loss *is* necessary to resolve your back pain. If you are unfamiliar with the Atkins diet, I encourage you to visit the website at www.AtkinsCenter.com. You will find the answers to most of your questions there.

Again, my patients who follow this low-carb, high-protein dietary plan stay healthy, have great checkups, and lose more weight even while consuming more calories than patients who follow low-fat diets. For patients with back pain, losing weight and keeping it off is necessary to help stop your pain, increase exercise, and allow you to cut back on medications.

The Zone Diet

Another popular high-protein, low-carbohydrate diet that has received a lot of attention over the past few years, as described in his book, is *The Zone Diet* by Dr. Barry Sears. Dr. Sears's theories involve balancing hormones and boosting metabolism with a specific ratio of foods that equals 40 percent carbohydrates, 30 percent protein, and 30 percent fat. This is now widely known as the "40-30-30 Plan."

The Zone diet does not forbid any foods, but severely restricts high-fat foods and certain carbohydrates such as grains, starches, and pastas. Fruits and vegetables are the favored source of carbohydrates in the Zone diet.

Protein is low fat only and portion controlled or about no thicker than the palm of your hand (see more discussion on portion sizes on page 50). The fats are good fats—monounsaturated fats such as olive oil, canola oil, almonds, macadamia nuts, and avocados (see page 57).

Dr. Sears teaches in his Zone diet to fill one-third of the plate with low-fat protein, and then pile the rest with vegetables and lentils, beans, whole grains, and most fruits. You may choose to add a monounsaturated source of fat such as olive oil or avocado. You can read more about the Zone diet online at www.drsears.com and decide if this plan fits your tastes and lifestyle.

Sugar Busters

The basic plan of Sugar Busters is to eat high-fiber vegetables, stone-ground whole grains, lean and trimmed meats, fish, and fruits. If you choose alcohol, you should drink red wine. As consumption of added sugars rose 22 percent between 1980 and 2000, reaching 31 teaspoons of added sugars per person per day, Sugar Busters and the other low-carb diets make great health sense.

The Sugar Busters authors say there are only a few things you cannot eat on the diet, including: potatoes, corn, white rice, bread from refined flour, beets, carrots, refined sugar, corn syrup, molasses, honey, sugared colas, and beer. Many people have successfully lost weight on Sugar Busters. To evaluate the diet and see if this fits your personal tastes, go online to www.sugarbusters.com.

Pain-Free Back Weight-Loss Tip #2:
Eat a Variety of Whole Foods

Once you've lost five or ten pounds, increase your intake of complex carbohydrates with fresh fruits and vegetables. I find that whole foods are a better choice for getting most vitamins and minerals rather than relying on supplements. With fruits you get specific vitamins, such as C, as well as all the essential nutrients necessary for immune function and energy. For instance, an orange is filled with vitamin C, carotene, and calcium. Oranges and other citrus fruits also help to ease your pain, as they are high in bioflavonoids, which come from plants and have strong antioxidant and anti-inflammatory properties. There is evidence that foods high in bioflavonoids enhance key enzyme reactions that lessen inflammation, which might help alleviate pain. Besides that, a fresh orange tastes great, especially after doing your Pain-Free Back Exercise Program.

Boost Antioxidants in Your Diet

Antioxidants help the body to heal quickly and prevent chronic illness. For example:

- Vitamin A is important in the synthesis of protein, the chief process of muscle growth.
- Vitamin C guards muscle cells from free radical damage and enhances recovery and growth (see page 56).
- Vitamin E protects the cell's membranes. Many metabolic processes occur in the body that are dependent upon healthy cell membranes, including the recuperation and growth of muscle cells.

Fresh whole fruits and vegetables are also high in antioxidants and phytochemicals. An antioxidant is a super nutrient that helps to repair cell damage and is vital to the body's resistance to infection. Phytochemicals are biologically active substances that give plants their color, flavor, and odor and protect against plant disease.

As you increase your intake of food, also increase your exercise program. Burning more calories than you take in will let you continue to lose weight as you eat more and still enjoy freedom from back pain and immobility. You might consider joining an organization such as Weight Watchers or Jennie Craig. Millions of men and women have had success with both of these fine groups.

Because strong muscles support your skeleton, keeping your muscles healthy with a varied diet of fresh fruits and vegetables and other foods high in antioxidants is important.

Pain-Free Back Weight-Loss Tip #3: Eat Lean Protein

If you choose to jump-start your diet with low-carb, high-protein foods, there are plenty of healthy protein choices from which to choose. Select leaner cuts of meat or poultry, since they are lower in fat and calories.

Eat more fish, which is high in protein and low in carbohydrates. You also get the benefit of omega-3 fatty acids when you eat fatty fish like salmon, sardines, tuna, and trout (see page 52). For instance, tuna is rich in omega-3 fatty acids (n-3 PUFA), eicosopentoic (EPA), and docosahexoic (DHA). These fatty acids are known to reduce inflammation and may

Stop Supersizing

It seems that when America went to supersizing meals, it was the same year America started its obesity epidemic. Being overweight increases our risk for back pain and other chronic ailments. Initially, it was thought that the supersizing of food was the result of creative marketing by fast-food restaurants hoping to sell more of it. However, an interesting study conducted by researchers at the University of North Carolina at Chapel Hill, published in the January 2003 *Journal of the American Medicine Association,* looked into foods such as hamburgers, burritos, tacos, french fries, sodas, ice cream, pie, cookies, and salty snacks and found that between the 1970s and the 1990s, the portion sizes increased—no matter if people ate these foods at home or at fast-food restaurants. Some of these findings:

- Homemade burgers beefed up to 8.4 ounces in 1996 from 5.7 ounces in 1977
- Fast-food hamburgers grew to 7.2 ounces in 1996 from 6.1 ounces in 1977
- At restaurants other than those serving fast food, hamburgers declined to 5 ounces in 1996 from 5.3 ounces in 1977.

It may not be just the type of food we're eating that is causing the obesity epidemic. The fact that we're eating such huge portions could say it all. The U.S. Department of Agriculture counts two to three ounces of cooked lean meat as a serving. And extra ounces mean extra calories.

Here are some helpful tips to shrink-wrap your serving portions:

- A cup of fruit should be no larger than your fist.
- One ounce of meat or cheese is about the same size as your thumb from base to tip.
- Three ounces of meat, fish, or poultry (a normal serving) is about the size of your palm.
- One to two ounces of nuts equals your cupped hand.
- Serve your meal on salad plates and pack away the large dinner plates.
- Store snack foods in tiny sandwich bags so you are sure you're eating no more than one portion.
- When ordering out, share your entree with your guest.
- Ask for a kid's meal or small size—not the supersize portion.
- Fill up on fresh green salads, whole fruits with the skin, and colorful vegetables instead of high-fat foods—breads, pasta, and desserts.

help ease back pain in some people. Vegetarians may prefer whole foods that contain another omega-3 fatty acid, alpha linolenic, including soybeans, canola oil, flaxseed, and nuts.

Be sure to include an array of soy foods, which are naturally low in calories, fat, and carbohydrates. Soy, the most complete vegetable protein, is also rich in vitamin E, fiber, calcium, magnesium, lecithin, riboflavin, thiamine, folic acid, iron, and essential fatty acids and should be a regular part of your Pain-Free Back Healthy Eating Plan.

Here are some of the high-protein choices I recommend to patients:

Lean Meat, Poultry, and Fish

Beef: USDA Select or Choice grades of lean beef trimmed of fat, such as round, sirloin, and flank steak; tenderloin; roast (rib, chuck, rump); steak (T-bone, porterhouse, cubed), ground round

Pork: lean pork, such as fresh ham; canned, cured, or boiled ham; Canadian bacon; tenderloin, center loin chop

Lamb: roast, chop, leg

Veal: lean chop, roast

Poultry: chicken, turkey (dark meat, no skin), chicken white meat (with skin), domestic duck or goose (well-drained of fat, no skin)

Fish: herring (uncreamed or smoked); oysters; salmon (fresh or canned); catfish; sardines (canned); tuna (canned in oil, drained); mackerel and other fatty fish

Game: goose (no skin); rabbit

Soy Protein

Edabame (beans
  in the pod)
Miso (paste)
Meat analogs (textured
  soy protein)
Soybeans
Soy cheese

Soy flour
Soy milk
Soy nuts
Tempeh
Tofu (soft; silken, firm, extra-firm)
Tofu (water-packed;
  firm or extra-firm)

Seeds and Nuts

Almonds
Almond butter
Macadamia nuts
Peanuts

Peanut butter
Pumpkin seeds
Sunflower seeds
Walnuts

Fish High in Omega-3 Fatty Acids

Anchovy   Mackerel
Bluefish   Atlantic Salmon
Capeline   Shad
Dogfish   Sardines
Tuna   Sturgeon
Atlantic Herring   Whitefish

Follow the Glycemic Index

Recent findings from Harvard Medical School indicate that you can use the glycemic index (GI) to choose carbohydrate foods that will have a relatively low impact on your blood sugar. The glycemic index is a numerical system that ranks carbohydrates on a scale of 0 to 100, according to their effect on blood glucose (sugar) levels. In the Harvard studies, scientists measured the amount of sugar that different foods released in the body right after they were ingested. Foods that gave a sugar "boost" appeared to increase weight gain and obesity, as well as added to the risk of getting heart disease and diabetes. These studies reported that foods pure in protein and fat (such as meat, chicken, and fish) have a glycemic index of zero. A baked potato has a glycemic index of 85. A food low on the glycemic index (meat, chicken, fish, soy products, and some vegetables) will cause a small rise in blood sugar; a food high on the glycemic index (the baked potato and other starchy foods) will trigger a more dramatic rise, which can cause an increase in appetite.

Choose foods low on the GI:
- Low-fat dairy
- Low-fat protein, tofu, nuts, and legumes
- Non-starchy vegetables
- Breakfast cereals based on wheat bran, barley, and oats
- Whole-grain breads made with whole seeds
- Barley, pasta, and rice instead of potatoes
- Vinegar and lemon juice dressing

Be cautious when selecting foods high on the GI:
- Potatoes
- Refined grains
- Sweets
- Vegetables high in starch (corn)
- Candy
- Pastries

Glycemic Index

Beans				
baby lima	32		Frosted Flakes	55
baked	43		Grapenuts	67
black	30		Grapenuts Flakes	80
brown	38		Life	66
butter	31		Muesli	60
chickpeas	33		NutriGrain	66
kidney	27		Oatmeal	49
lentil	30		Oatmeal (quick)	66
navy	38		Puffed Wheat	74
pinto	42		Puffed Rice	90
red lentils	27		Rice Bran	19
split peas	32		Rice Chex	89
soy	18		Rice Krispies	82
			Shredded Wheat	69
Breads			Special K	54
bagel	72		Swiss Muesli	60
croissant	67		Team	82
Kaiser roll	73		Total	76
pita	57			
pumpernickel	49		**Cookies**	
rye	64		graham crackers	74
rye, dark	76		oatmeal	55
rye, whole	50		shortbread	64
white	72		Vanilla Wafers	77
whole wheat	72			
waffles	76		**Crackers**	
			rice cakes	82
Cereals			rye	63
All Bran	44		wheat thins	67
Bran Chex	58		water crackers	78
Cheerios	74			
Corn Bran	75		**Desserts**	
Corn Chex	83		angel food cake	67
Cornflakes	83		banana bread	47
Cream of Wheat	66		blueberry muffin	59
Crispix	87		bran muffin	60
			pound cake	54

Glycemic Index *(continued)*

Desserts *(continued)*

sponge cake	46

Fruit

apple	38
apricot, canned	64
apricot, dried	30
apricot jam	55
banana	62
banana, unripe	30
cantaloupe	65
cherries	22
fruit cocktail	55
grapefruit	25
grapes	43
kiwi	52
mango	55
orange	43
papaya	58
peach	42
pear	36
pineapple	66
plum	24
raisins	64
strawberries	32
strawberry jam	51
watermelon	72

Grains

barley	22
brown rice	59
buckwheat	54
bulgur	47
cornmeal	68
couscous	65
hominy	40
millet	75

rice, instant	91
rice, parboiled	47
rye	34
sweet corn	55
wheat, whole	41
white rice	88

Juices

apple	41
grapefruit	48
orange	55
pineapple	46

Milk Products

chocolate milk	34
ice cream	50
milk	34
pudding	43
soy milk	31
yogurt	38

Pasta

brown rice pasta	92
gnocchi	68
linguine, durum	50
macaroni	46
macaroni and cheese	64
spaghetti	40
vermicelli	35

Sweets

honey	58
jelly beans	80
Life Savers	70
M&M's Choc. Peanut	33
Skittles	70
Snickers	41

Pain-Free Back Weight-Loss Tip #4:
Fill Up on High-Fiber Complex Carbohydrates
You can enhance the weight-loss benefits of a low-carb, high-protein diet, or any weight-loss plan for that matter, if you eat high-fiber complex carbs, including fresh fruits, vegetables, legumes, and whole grains. Because fiber coats the stomach lining, it delays stomach emptying and slows digestion and sugar absorption after a meal, reducing the amount of insulin needed. Again, this insulin response is what triggers hunger pangs—something you want to squelch when you're trying to lose weight.

I tell my patients to eat from the rainbow, selecting different colors of fruits and vegetables to ensure optimal nutrition. These colorful, high-fiber complex carbs are filled with phytochemicals, bioflavinoids, carotenoids such as isoflavones, lycopene, and polyphenols, and other compounds that we know may reduce the risk of serious chronic illness.

Here are some of the high-fiber complex carbohydrates I recommend to patients:

Vegetables	Fresh Fruits
Artichokes	Apples
Asparagus	Apricots
Beans	Avocados
Broccoli	Bananas
Brussels sprouts	Blackberries
Cabbages	Blueberries
Carrots	Cantaloupes
Celery	Cherries
Cucumbers	Grapefruits
Eggplants	Honeydew melons
Lentils	Kiwi fruits
Lettuce (dark green)	Lemons
Mushrooms	Limes
Onions	Oranges
Peas	Pineapples
Red and green peppers	Raspberries
Spinach	Strawberries
Squash	Tangerines
Zucchini	Tomatoes

Whole Grains

Barley	Millet
Bulgur	Oats
Bran	Polenta
Brown rice	Quinoa
Couscous	Whole grain bread and pasta

Up Your C's

Vitamin C, a water-soluble vitamin, is plentiful in fresh fruits and vegetables. This key antioxidant helps to maintain the strength of collagen (an important part of the cartilage that cushions the joints), ligaments, and tendons and can block the effect of inflammatory substances, which can lead to pain and destruction in the body. Studies show that vitamin C inhibits the breakdown of cartilage and may be beneficial to those with back pain from osteoarthritis, since the cartilage is often adversely affected.

You can get enough vitamin C by eating five servings of fresh fruits and vegetables daily, including any of the following: broccoli, cauliflower, peppers, kale, Brussels sprouts, cabbage, citrus fruit, melons, asparagus, avocado, kohlrabi, mustard greens, tomato, and watercress. Supplementation with a vitamin C tablet may be advised if your diet is inadequate, so ask your doctor if you are concerned.

Fiber Content of Food (Listed from highest to lowest)

1. Whole grains, including cooked cereals and breads from barley, oats, buckwheat, rice, rye, quinoa, spelt, wheat, and corn (processed grains and bread made with flour don't count).
2. Legumes—lentils, peas, and beans (including refried, no-fat garbanzos on salads and soy beans).
3. Nuts, seeds, and dried fruits. High in calories—eat in moderation.
4. Root vegetables, including yams, carrots, beets, and potatoes.
5. Other vegetables, including broccoli, green beans, and leafy greens.
6. Fruit, including berries, pears, apples, and prunes (juice has *no* fiber).
7. Lettuce, cabbage, and celery.
8. Meat, chicken, milk, cheese, and eggs (these contain no fiber).

Fats Are Not the Dieter's Enemy!

Say YES to Good Fat:

• **Monounsaturated fat** is good fat. It comes from oils that are liquid at room temperature or, better still, plant foods (avocados, nuts, peanut oil, canola oil, tahini, olives, fish). Research suggests that these fats may actually reduce your LDL ("bad") cholesterol level without lowering the HDL ("good") cholesterol, helping to reduce your risk of cardiovascular disease.

• **Omega-3 fats** are found in fatty fish (anchovy, mackerel, salmon, sardines, shad, and tuna), flaxseed, and nuts. Studies show that omega-3 fats reduce the risk of blood clots and abnormal heart rhythms and improve blood cholesterol and triglycerides. Another type of omega-3 fatty acid is alpha-linolenic acid, which is found in flaxseed, canola and soybean oils, walnuts, and dark green leafy vegetables.

• **Polyunsaturated fat** comes from oils that are liquid or soft at room temperature, including corn, safflower, sesame, soybean, and sunflower oils. While polyunsaturated fat lowers LDL or "bad" cholesterol, it also lowers your HDL or "good" cholesterol, which you want to raise. (**Caution:** some findings indicate that a diet high in polyunsaturated vegetable oils encourages the synthesis of *pro-inflammatory* prostaglandins, the group of hormones that intensify the inflammatory response. That's why choosing more omega-3 fatty acids—salmon, sardines, walnuts, flaxseeds or oil, and soy foods—that increase the production of *inhibitory* prostaglandins is important in your daily diet.)

Say NO to Bad Fat:

• **Cholesterol** is found in meat, dairy, and egg yolks. Food cholesterol increases the blood cholesterol, adding to your risk of heart disease.

• **Saturated fat** comes from animal sources, whole milk dairy products, and some oils. Saturated fat is found in red meat, butter, cheeses, luncheon meats, cocoa butter, coconut oil, palm oil, and cream.

• **Hydrogenated fat** is made during a chemical process called hydrogenation, in which naturally unsaturated liquid oil changes into a solid and more saturated form. The greater the amount of hydrogenation, the more saturated the fat becomes, which can raise your blood cholesterol levels.

- **Trans fats** are formed when unsaturated vegetable oils are hydrogenated to make them solid at room temperature (stick margarine). In the ongoing National Institutes of Health Nurses Health Study, researchers found that among 80,000 women aged 34 to 59, trans fats greatly increased the risk for coronary heart disease. In these findings, researchers reported that each 2 percent increase in trans fat calories raised the women's coronary risk by 93 percent. Other high trans fat foods include fried foods, snack and fast-food products, commercial breads, crackers, pastries, and many processed foods.

Nuts and "Good" Fat

Nuts are a super source of vitamin E and are loaded with "good" fat. But nuts are also high in calories. For instance, you only get two teaspoons of almonds for 100 calories. Include nuts in your diet, but also keep track of how many you eat.

Nut	Calories per Ounce	% Saturated Fat	% Mono- unsaturated Fat	% Poly- unsaturated Fat
Almonds	166.41	9.9	67.6	22.5
Macadamias	199.02	15.3	82.4	2.3
Peanuts	165.5	14.9	52.2	32.9
Soy nuts	128.4	15.8	23.7	60.5
Walnuts	172.1	6.8	23.3	69.9

Pain-Free Back Weight-Loss Tip #5:
Eliminate Junk Food from Your Kitchen

You've got to clean out your kitchen if you're going to lose weight. After all, who can resist eating some chips or homemade cookies while watching TV at night? Not many of us! Not having tempting foods around will help you to stay compliant to your weight-loss plan and see faster results in reduced pain.

No matter which weight-loss plan you choose, go through your refrigerator and cupboards and get rid of *any foods* that will cause you to overeat or binge eat. Then make an itemized shopping list to buy *only those foods* allowed in your food plan, using the lists in this step.

When you shop for groceries, follow the perimeter of the grocery store where the fresh foods are and avoid the displays and inner aisles (that's generally where the junk and packaged foods are). Foods I want you to keep stocked in your kitchen include the following:

- Fat-free milk, yogurt, and cheese
- Eggs/egg substitutes
- White-meat chicken or turkey
- Soy products
- Fish and shellfish
- Dried peas and beans
- Fresh, frozen, and canned fruits and vegetables
- Seeds and nuts
- Sugarfree gelatin, drinks, and gum
- Green and black tea

Pain-Free Back Weight-Loss Tip #6: Eat Frequently
It's interesting that when most of us decide to lose weight, we immediately *stop* eating. Researchers now know that the best way to maintain a normal weight is to stop dieting and eat more frequently with mini-meals.

Dieting, as we've done it previously, greatly restricts calories and nutritious foods causing you to feel deprived and resulting in rebound bingeing or overeating. Eating healthful foods *more frequently* will boost your metabolism and productivity. Research has found that people who eat two meals or less during the day have a slower metabolic rate (the speed at which your body burns calories, a rate we all want to go faster) versus those who eat three or more times a day. Eating frequently will also keep your blood glucose constant, which helps you to not feel irritable or overly hungry. In addition, here is another bonus: when you eat frequently, there is an increase in your metabolic rate. A faster metabolism helps to burn calories and boosts weight loss.

Rules for Eating Mini-Meals

- Break your daily food intake into five or six mini-meals.
- Space these meals every three to four hours throughout the day.
- Allow about 300 to 400 calories per meal, depending on your total caloric goal.

Super Nutrients That Keep Bones Strong

Not only is weight loss vital for resolving back pain, but eating specific foods and nutrients can keep your bones strong and prevent osteoporosis. Review the following vitamins and minerals and make sure you get the recommended dietary allowance (RDA).

Calcium

Osteoporosis (loss of bone density) is a common cause of back pain and results in fractures of the vertebrae (and other bones). Most men and women aren't even aware that they have osteoporosis until they break a bone and live with the excruciating pain. Calcium, the most abundant mineral in the body, plays a vital role in preventing osteoporosis since it helps to keep bones and teeth strong. But calcium must be replenished daily through dietary measures or supplementation, otherwise your body will be deficient.

Although the daily calcium recommendation for adults is approximately 1,000 to 1,200 milligrams (higher for pregnant and lactating women, postmenopausal women, and elderly men and women), the average adult gets only two-thirds to three-quarters of that amount. Some studies reveal that 80 percent of American women do not get adequate amounts of this bone-strengthening mineral. For example, extreme dieting can result in loss of bone density if you aren't ingesting adequate calcium. A low calcium intake during adolescence also affects bone density, as can certain medications and other risk factors (see page 176). But getting adequate calcium through foods or supplements is something you can do each day to prevent back pain from fractures.

Although the risk of bone fractures increases with age, new findings presented at the 51st annual meeting of the American College of Obstetricians and Gynecologists in May 2003 suggest that many women develop dangerously low bone mass and fractures even during the first years after menopause. Researchers said that in examinations of almost 90,000 women between the ages of 50 and 64, almost one-third had bone mass low enough to put them at a higher risk of fracture. They concluded that doctors need to focus on the problem of low bone mass and fracture in their younger postmenopausal patients, as well as in older women. In the studies, younger women had an increased risk of fracture if they had low bone mass, had experienced a fracture after age 45, had generally poor health, and if their mothers had also experienced bone fractures in old age.

Juice It!

Studies have found that drinking juices fortified with calcium may be an even better way to get calcium than drinking milk. One revealing study, reported in the June 1996 issue of the *Journal of the American College of Nutrition,* concluded that while people could absorb only about 25 to 30 percent of the calcium in milk, they could absorb about 36 percent of the calcium in fortified orange juice and 42 percent in the calcium-enriched apple juice.

It appears that the body's ability to absorb the calcium in foods is related to other substances that are present besides calcium. In this particular study, it was found that the type and amounts of sugar, and the acid content of the drink, affected how calcium was absorbed by the body.

Usually, dietary calcium can reach the recommended amounts simply by including three or four servings of calcium-rich foods each day. Milk, cheese, and yogurt are easy sources and have an added benefit in that they contain lactose, which enhances calcium absorption. If you are watching your weight, select low-fat milk and by-products. Other sources of calcium include salmon with bones, sardines, calcium-enriched juices and other food products, soy foods, and green leafy vegetables. Nevertheless, keep in mind that you have eat a lot of non-dairy foods to get your calcium because it's not as easily absorbed by your body, as it is in

---

10 Non-Dairy Calcium-Rich Foods

1. Beans (pinto, black, white)
2. Broccoli
3. Dry roasted almonds
4. Tofu and soy products
5. Figs
6. Greens (collards, kale, spinach)
7. Rhubarb
8. Salmon with bones
9. Pink canned salmon, canned shrimp
10. Fortified juices and cereals

Calcium Superstars

500 milligrams
8.5 ounces of cheese-filled manicotti
Instant breakfast drink made with 1 cup low-fat milk
1 cup calcium-fortified milk
1 fruited yogurt smoothie with ¼ cup powdered skim milk added
1 small cheese pizza

400 milligrams
8 medium sardines, canned with bones
8 ounces of nonfat yogurt
12 ounces of enchiladas with cheese
4 buckwheat pancakes, 4-inch diameter
1 average chocolate milkshake

300 milligrams
Orange juice with added calcium
Calcium-fortified cereal with ½ cup milk
Cream of broccoli soup made with milk and cheese
1 ¼ cups black beans
1 cup of scalloped potatoes with cheese

200 milligrams
½ cup instant pudding made with milk
1 ounce American cheese
1 cup steamed kale
1 cup macaroni and cheese

dairy foods. For instance, you'd need to consume 8 cups of spinach, nearly 5 cups of red beans, or 2½ cups of broccoli to get the same amount of calcium absorbed from one cup of milk.

While getting calcium from food is preferable because of the other vitamins and minerals present, you can also get your daily calcium requirement from supplements, particularly those made from calcium carbonate or citrate.

Vitamin D
Although vitamin D is usually categorized as a fat-soluble vitamin, it actually functions as a hormone in the body. Vitamin D helps to activate

calcium and phosphorus (another key mineral for keeping bones strong) in the bloodstream. When the body is depleted of vitamin D or has an insufficient supply, the blood levels of calcium and phosphorus plummet as well. Your body turns to the bones for replenishing this mineral. Loss of the minerals calcium and phosphorus is directly correlated to osteoporosis and a host of other bone-weakening problems that increases your risk of back injury and pain. New findings from Boston University show that vitamin D is an important nutrient for multiple facets of health—including insulin function, cancer prevention (especially of the breast/colon/prostate), and cardiovascular health.

Although younger adults get plenty of sunlight throughout the day to keep this vitamin in check, many middle-aged and older adults may have a problem. In comprehensive studies at the New England Medical Center, researchers concluded that aging reduces the skin's capability to make use of sunlight to manufacture vitamin D. Consequently, daily vitamin D supplements of 800 IU (International Units) per day at age sixty-five to seventy are suggested. Some experts suggest that men and women over fifty take 800 IU of vitamin D year-round.

The usual recommended dietary allowance (RDA) for vitamin D is 400 IU. Along with sunlight, you can also obtain this bone-strengthening vitamin from food sources, such as halibut-liver oil, herring, cod-liver oil, mackerel, salmon, tuna, fortified milk, and fortified cereals. If you are not getting adequate amounts, vitamin D supplements should seriously be considered.

Vitamin K
Vitamin K is still another vitamin that plays a vital role in calcium absorption and an indirect role in preventing bone loss with osteoporosis. The RDA for this vitamin is 65 to 80 micrograms. The best food sources include green leafy vegetables, soybean oil, broccoli, alfalfa, cooked spinach, and fish oil.

Magnesium
Magnesium has a key function in numerous biochemical reactions that are necessary for bone strength and metabolism. This mineral regulates active calcium transport and might play a role in stopping bone fractures. Some findings reveal that many older women with osteoporosis are lacking in magnesium, even when their calcium levels are adequate.

About 60 percent of dietary magnesium is stored in the bones, while muscle and other tissues use the rest. The recommended dosages of magnesium range from 280 milligrams for women and 350 milligrams for men. A good rule of thumb is to take *one milligram of magnesium for every two milligrams of calcium*.

Food sources of magnesium include cereals, nuts, sunflower seeds, tofu, and dairy products; bananas, pineapples, plantains, raisins, artichokes, avocados, lima beans, spinach, okra, beet greens; oysters, halibut, mackerel, grouper, cod, and sole.

Boron

Boron, another mineral plentiful in fruits and vegetables, appears to play an active role in the metabolism of calcium and bone development.

Soy Keeps Bones Strong

Some comprehensive studies show that adding one serving a day of soybeans (or soy by-product) to your diet may actually increase bone strength. One study was done at the University of Illinois on sixty-six postmenopausal women who were not taking hormone replacements. The group of women who took 90 milligrams of isoflavones a day for six months increased their bone density by 3 percent, as well as the bone mineral content of the lumbar spine. (The lumbar spine is the small of the back and is prone to fractures after menopause.) Though the increase was small, it is significant, and offers tremendous hope to women who cannot do hormone replacement therapy at menopause.

Isoflavones are plant compounds that mimic estrogen, although isoflavones are a lot weaker than human estrogen (about five hundred to one thousand times weaker than the body's hormone). Many revealing studies have found that isoflavones have some of the actions of estrogen in the body. In osteoporosis research, isoflavones have been shown to inhibit bone breakdown in animals because of their estrogen-like actions. Studies show that eating animal protein can weaken bones as it causes the body to remove calcium quicker. In a breakthrough study, researchers found that those who ate soy protein instead of animal protein lost 50 percent less calcium in the urine, thus helping to keep bones dense and strong. Because Japanese women have half the rate of hip fractures as women in the United States, preliminary studies suggest that soy may be the key factor in helping to retain bone mass.

Although still controversial, research by the U.S. Department of Agriculture indicates that boron increases estrogen levels in the blood. As such, some researchers believe that this mineral might enhance estrogen's effects in women using estrogen replacement therapy (ERT), and it may be helpful to retain calcium and magnesium.

Although there is no established recommendation for boron, you can get this mineral in plentiful amounts in vegetables, legumes (dried beans and peas), dried fruits, seeds, and nuts. Avoid taking mega-doses with supplements since there can be side effects such as headaches.

Phosphorus

Phosphorus is a key mineral in almost all chemical reactions in the body, and it also works side by side with calcium to build strong bones and teeth. The RDA for phosphorus is 800 milligrams for adults (1,200 milligrams for pregnant and lactating women). You can find phosphorus in fish, poultry, meats, grains, eggs, seeds, and nuts.

Manganese

Manganese, an antioxidant, may also be important in preventing osteoporosis because it offers a possible tie-in with bone and connective tissue development. The recommended intake of this trace element is 2.5 to 5 milligrams daily. Food sources rich in manganese include grains and grain products, nuts, legumes, seeds, and green leafy vegetables.

More Super Nutrients to Ease Back Pain

Breakthrough studies are strong on the ties between nutrition, food, and a healthy immune system. In fact, deficiencies of single nutrients can result in altered immune responses, which have been observed even when the deficiency is relatively mild. It seems as if almost weekly we see news about specific foods and their ties to chronic pain. What is so special about these foods? Scientists have studied them individually to try to determine how they work to end pain.

Take soy, for example. Not only does dietary soy help to keep bones strong, it may help to soothe your pain. In a study presented at the 2002 annual meeting of the American Pain Society in Baltimore, Maryland, researchers from Johns Hopkins suggested that a diet rich in soy may help ease chronic pain caused by inflammation and swelling (back pain falls into this category).

In the study, researchers fed a soy-based diet to rats with chronic inflammation-type pain. These same scientists concluded that rats that were fed soy were better able to withstand heat when it was applied to their injured foot, and they had significantly less swelling than did rats fed milk. Of course, this is preliminary—and it's about rats, not humans. Still, I believe that it's no coincidence that what we eat—or don't eat—can affect our health, immune function, and healing. Here are some foods and nutrients that have been recognized as vital for helping to prevent pain.

Bananas

Bananas have vitamin B_6 and tryptophan—both important for promoting a sense of calmness when life's stressors cause you to feel tense. Vitamin B_6 is important for the synthesis of serotonin and dopamine, neurotransmitters that are necessary for healthy nerve cell communication. Tryptophan is an amino acid that stimulates serotonin, the neurotransmitter that has a calming effect on the body. Enjoy a banana when tension begins to result in a nagging backache, and see if this nutrient combo might help.

Berries

Dark berries (blueberries, blackberries, cherries, and raspberries) are helpful in easing pain because they contain anthocyanidins, which sweep out harmful free-radical molecules. The vitamin C in berries helps to strengthen the immune system and is important in producing connective tissue, especially collagen.

Cherries

Cherries contain the compound cyanidin, which is thought to block inflammatory enzymes.

Green Tea

Sipping green tea throughout the day may give unexpected health benefits. Tea is full of catechins, complex organic molecules that may help to reduce pain and boost weight loss. Overall, green tea has the most catechins per cup—about 30 to 40 percent of dry matter; black tea, which is more popular in America, has considerably less—about 5 to 10 percent of dry matter. In a study presented at the Society of Critical Care Medicine, researchers found that green tea may help block the arthritis-inflammatory response.

Green tea contains a type of polyphenol known as epigallocatechin-3-gallate, or EGCG that inhibits the expression of the interleukin-8 gene, which is a substance that signals the body's white blood cells and other mediators to promote inflammation. A cup of green tea may provide 10 to 40 milligrams of polyphenols and has antioxidant activity greater than a serving of broccoli, spinach, or strawberries. Researchers theorize that "more may be better" when it comes to drinking green tea to help reduce pain and stiffness.

Another recent study of more than 1,200 older British women, published in the April 2000 *American Journal of Nutrition*, concluded that those who drank the most tea (four or more cups a day) had higher bone-density levels in their spines and hips than those who drank less tea or no tea at all. Because higher bone-mineral density generally means a lower risk of fracture (from falling, for example), tea had a definite protective effect for these women. A recent study of more than a thousand men and women in China found the same result. In this study, published in the October 2002 issue of the *Archives of Internal Medicine*, study participants who drank the most tea had the highest bone-mineral density levels—and the longer they had been drinking tea on a regular basis, the higher their levels were.

Studies are just coming in on the thermogenic properties of certain foods, and green tea may be at the top of the list. In a study published in June 1999 in the *American Journal of Clinical Nutrition*, researchers found that capsules containing green tea extract made metabolisms run faster so they burned up more fat. This is very preliminary, but it shows the direction food science is heading, proving that maybe we are what we eat after all!

Oranges

Oranges have the flavonoid nobiletin, which may have an anti-inflammatory action. Hesperidin, another flavonoid, is found in the thin, orange portion of the citrus peel. Hesperidin may also reduce inflammation.

Peppers

Sweet bell peppers, as well as spicy chili peppers, have capsaicin, which is the fiery phytochemical capsaicin. Capsaicin reduces levels of substance P, the compound in the body that triggers inflammation and pain impulses from the central nervous system. It is thought that this pain-relieving phytochemical triggers the body to release endorphins, nature's own opiates. Red peppers are also filled with salicylates, which are aspirin-like compounds.

Pineapple

For years, I've recommended pineapple to athletes to help heal sports injuries. The reason is bromelain, the key enzyme in pineapple that helps reduce inflammation. Some studies show that bromelain enzymes can help reduce pain in osteoarthritis. Pineapple also has manganese, a bone-building mineral, and vitamin C, which helps to strengthen collagen.

Your Pain-Free Back Healthy Eating Plan Rx

I realize that you cannot lose that twenty pounds overnight—after all, it took you years to add those pounds to your body. But you can start today

"B" Pain-Free

Some new research points to the use of B vitamins in the treatment of chronic pain, particularly nocioceptive pain, which comes from sprains, fractures, bumps, bruises, inflammation from infection or arthritic dis-order, and myofascial pain—abnormal muscle stresses. Previous studies explored the possibility that the analgesic and inflammatory effects of vitamin B_1 (thiamin), B_6 (pyridoxine), and B_{12} (cyanocobalamin) might reduce inflammation. The new findings, presented at the American Physiological Society Conference, Experimental Biology 2003, in San Diego, California, concluded that some B vitamins, such as thiamin (B_1), pyridoxine (B_6), and cyanocobalamin (B_{12}) may be clinically effective in treating various painful conditions such as lumbago, sciatica, and other types of pain by acting as an analgesic (pain reliever).

Add Avocados

While you are learning about how foods can decrease inflammation and pain, add avocados to your list. These nutrient-dense foods have the highest fiber content of any fruit (yes, avocado is a fruit!) and are filled with vitamins C and E, folic acid, magnesium, and potassium. Sixty percent of the fat in an avocado is monounsaturated, and there is no saturated fat or cholesterol. For those on the low-carb diet, avocados are relatively low in carbohydrates, too, with 14 carbs per whole avo-cado and 10 grams of fiber.

Pain Busters

In a few studies, patients reported feeling less pain and stiffness by adding certain foods to their diets. If you are not allergic to these foods, it would not hurt to try them and find out if they give benefit.

- Garlic, onions, and cabbage to increase sulfur content. Sulfur aids in reducing inflammation
- Cherries, blackberries, and blueberries to boost cartilage formation and prevent cartilage destruction
- Celery, parsley, apples, whole grains, alfalfa, ginger, and licorice to balance immune function

---

by cleaning out your kitchen and removing unhealthy snacks and junk food. Make up a grocery list of healthful foods and shop the perimeter of the grocery store for fresh whole foods. In addition, begin today to keep an ongoing record of the foods you eat in your Pain-Free Back Diary. By using these starting suggestions, you'll have an idea of your current eating habits and will not be tempted to indulge in high-calorie junk or fast foods.

If you need more information on weight loss, talk to your doctor or a registered dietitian. Also, ask your spouse, another family member, or a friend to join your diet with you, as you did with the Pain-Free Back Exercise Program in Step 1. Compliance to a weight-loss plan is much easier when you have someone to share the ups and downs with, either by telephone, e-mail, or in person.

Use this checklist to implement each suggestion in Step 2 in your daily routine.

Pain-Free Back Healthy Eating Plan Rx

____ Find your ideal weight and write it down in your Pain-Free Back Diary.

____ Calculate the calories needed to lose weight and maintain an ideal weight.

____ Review the new low-carb, high-protein diets to see if any of them will help you get started.

____ Watch your portion sizes.

____ Clean out your kitchen pantry and refrigerator.

___ Eat lean protein including meat, poultry, fish, soy products, nuts, and seeds.

___ Eat a variety of whole foods.

___ Include high-fiber complex carbohydrates.

___ Avoid supersizing meals.

___ Say YES to good fat; say NO to bad fat.

___ Eat frequently.

___ Keep an ongoing journal of what you eat.

___ Boost bone strength with the vitamins and minerals.

___ Reduce inflammation and pain with the nutrients.

___ Diet with a friend.

Back to Nature

From valerian to St. John's wort, from glucosamine to fish oil, from SAMe to 5-HTP, dietary supplements are a billion-dollar business in America today. Most supermarket shelves resemble a natural pharmacy, stocked with rows and rows of herbal therapies, vitamins, minerals, natural enzymes, organ tissues, metabolites, extracts, or concentrates, and more. This "back to nature" trend represents the increasing demand by millions of Americans who want to take charge of their health and healing with complementary and alternative medicine (CAM) therapies.

If used appropriately, CAM modalities can boost your self-efficacy, and we doctors know that feeling in control of your health is essential for wellness. Proponents of complementary and alternative treatments claim that these nondrug interventions might allow you to take less medication, have fewer laboratory tests and surgeries, and be a proactive participant in self-care. Still, if used haphazardly, some complementary and alternative medicines are toxic and can interact with other medications you are taking. As a few have learned, taking the wrong dietary supplement might add to your health problems if there is an adverse reaction.

Forty-seven-year-old Teresa became a believer in complementary and alternative medicines after taking glucosamine, an over-the-counter dietary supplement for spinal arthritis pain, and valerian, an herb that has calming and sedating properties.

Teresa's high-stress sales job and weekly airline travel kept her in a constant state of tension, making it difficult to sleep in hotels during her business trips. To control her stress and anxiety, she was taking two prescription medications and a sleep preparation that left her feeling tired and dull. When Terri's dismal sales reports began to reflect her anxiety and fatigue, a coworker mentioned that she might get relief with natural dietary supplements such as valerian for insomnia and glucosamine to reduce her arthritis and back pain.

Before taking these popular supplements, Teresa did some research and talked with her primary physician to make sure they were safe. She also investigated meditation and yoga for stress reduction, and signed up for an aquatics class and yoga sessions at the Y.

Just as she was committed to her career success, Teresa was loyal to her natural therapy regimen. And within eight weeks, she felt like a new

---

Pain-Free Back Diary

Keeping track of your natural dietary supplements is important. As you did in Steps 1 and 2, continue to use your Pain-Free Back Diary or PDA (see page 4) to keep track of your progress in Step 3. Write down all complementary and alternative medicines, so you and your doctor have an accurate record. Make an appointment with your physician(s) to talk about CAM therapies. Let your doctor(s) know which therapies you are using, including vitamin and mineral supplements. Before you take anything that is not prescribed, make sure the supplements will not interact with prescribed or over-the-counter medications. Also, check for toxicity to minimize possible problems.

Before taking the supplements discussed in this step, talk to your doctor or pharmacist about possible side effects or herb-drug interactions. Herbal therapies are not recommended for pregnant women, children, the elderly, or those with compromised immune systems. In addition, some herbs have sedative or blood-thinning qualities, which may dangerously interact with NSAIDs or other pain medications. Others may cause gastrointestinal upset if taken in large doses.

No herb or pharmaceutical is 100 percent safe and effective. In 2001 some forty people died from the misuse of herbs. Still, this number does not begin to approach the percentage of casualties caused by FDA-approved drugs. Whether natural dietary supplement or FDA-approved pharmaceuticals, always know that there will be some side effects, along with the positive healing effects. A good website that keeps consumers informed about dietary supplements that may be unsafe or recalled is www.fda.gov/medwatch/safety.htm. Check this site periodically to make sure you are taking safe supplements.

Definition of a Dietary Supplement

According to the Food and Drug Administration (FDA), in order for an ingredient of a dietary supplement to be a "dietary ingredient," it must be one or any combination of the following substances:

- Vitamin
- Mineral
- Herb or other botanical
- Amino acid
- Substance that supplements the diet by increasing the total dietary intake
- Extract (solution of essential constituents)

---

person. She was sleeping well at night, even during travel, and her back pain had lessened dramatically. Because of less pain, Teresa had greater energy and became increasingly more active. She started walking the concourses of the airport instead of riding in the shuttle. She also took advantage of the exercise room and warm Jacuzzi in hotels during her travels. This boost in aerobic activity resulted in weight loss, stronger muscles, and reduced stress and muscle tension. Teresa began to sleep soundly at night and soon she stopped taking the valerian to relax during the evenings. She continued with the glucosamine, since it greatly eased her arthritis pain.

Today, Teresa continues to check in with her medical doctor, but remains a firm believer in using complementary and alternative medicines and positive lifestyle changes to resolve health problems.

From Ancient Days to New Age

The belief in complementary and alternative treatments is not a new revelation. The Chinese have used herbs for centuries to treat and cure a host of medical problems; Ayurvedic medicine, which focuses on balancing the body using such methods as meditation, herbs and minerals, and yoga go back four thousand years in India's rich history; and massage therapies, which relieve stress and tension through manual touch and manipulation go back to the beginning of time. Even in Western or conventional medicine, more than half of drugs commonly used today are either plant products or phytochemicals that were initially isolated from botanical material and are now synthesized by chemical processing techniques.

From Aristotle's time to the present, medical literature reveals anecdotal material documenting the use of unconventional treatments, as well as the intimate connection between mind, body, and spirit. Yet, it was not until the mid-sixties that Americans became intrigued with alternative medicine. At that time, the Vietnam War was invoking major changes in American society, particularly the exposure to Eastern Asian culture, including medical practices used there. This exposure, along with the increasing costs of our nation's health care, began to fuel the rapid adoption of complementary and alternative therapies in the United States.

Today, complementary and alternative medicines are commonplace. A 2001 national survey on the use of dietary supplements, the Dietary Supplement Barometer Survey, found that the majority of Americans believes in supplements and takes them on a regular basis. A market research report, by Kalorama Information, "The U.S. Market for Vitamins, Supplements, and Minerals," indicates that 30 million consumers use herbal remedies instead of over-the-counter (OTC) treatments, and an additional 19 million combine herbs and OTC remedies to treat their health problems.

Establishing the Effectiveness of CAM

In response to the tremendous demand for natural therapies for healing, Congress formed the National Center for Complementary and Alternative Medicine (NCCAM) as part of the National Institutes of Health (NIH) to help appraise alternative medical treatments and establish their effectiveness. This organization is now creating safe guidelines to help people choose appropriate alternative and complementary therapies.

The outlook for complementary and alternative medicine is remarkably optimistic, and we are gaining a better understanding of these nonstandard treatments and how they can increase health and prevent disease. Here are just a few of the breakthrough studies now being reported:

• In a 2000 study published in the *American Journal of Medicine*, a team of German researchers conducted a four-week clinical trial designed to compare the effectiveness and safety of two different dosages of white willow (*Salix*), also called white-willow bark or willow bark, for alleviating flare-ups of low back pain. Results showed that both the high and low doses of afforded significantly more pain relief than placebo, but the higher dose of willow bark (240 mg/day) was significantly more effective than either the low-dose treatment or the placebo.

According to the study, 39 percent of participants in the high-dose willow bark group were pain-free during the final week of treatment as compared to 21 percent of the low-dose group and only 6 percent of the placebo group.

• In a randomized double-blind study involving 240 patients over six weeks, German researchers concluded that hypericum (St. John's wort) was as effective as the selective serotonin reuptake inhibitors (SSRIs) such as Prozac, but without any serious side effects. In the study, published in the July 2000 issue of the *International Clinical Psychopharmacology*, 114 participants took 20 milligrams of fluoxetine (Prozac) twice daily; 128 participants took hypericum extract (St. John's wort) at a dose of 250 milligrams twice daily. All patients were evaluated by psychiatrists using the Hamilton Depression Scale (HAM-D), a common screening test used to assess depression symptoms. (Minor depression is a common but significant disorder that may impair functioning and quality of life. It is also a serious risk factor for major depression.)

After six weeks of treatment, improvement was nearly identical in the two groups. However, researchers found that safety of treatment was far superior for St. John's wort, since participants reported fewer and less serious side effects. Of all the side effects, the fluoxetine (Prozac) group reported far more serious symptoms, such as "dizziness, tiredness, anxiety, and erectile dysfunction." A few participants in the St. John's wort group reported mild gastrointestinal complaints.

The researchers concluded that St. John's wort clearly is superior as the medication of choice for mild to moderate depression in both efficacy and safety, particularly in situations where treatment is a choice between fluoxetine and hypericum.

• According to a study published in the May 2000 issue of the *Journal of the Royal Society of Medicine*, researchers at the University of Plymouth in England applied stinging nettle leaves to the hands of twenty-seven arthritis sufferers. After one week, the stinging nettles not only significantly reduced pain but the level of that pain stayed lower through most of the treatment. The nettles contain serotonin and histamine, both neurotransmitters that affect pain perception and transmission at the nerve endings.

• Researchers compared the effectiveness of willow bark with a COX-2 inhibitor (a COX-2 NSAID, discussed on page 194) in a study published in the *British Journal of Rheumatology*. Both groups reported a decrease in pain. Researchers concluded that there was no significant difference in effectiveness between the two treatments at the doses chosen, but treatment with white willow bark was about 40 percent less expensive.

• New evidence published in the January 2001 issue of *The Lancet*, a prominent British medical journal, suggested that glucosamine might slow the progression of osteoarthritis. In the study, 212 people with osteoarthritis were randomly selected to receive either 1,500 milligrams of glucosamine each day or a placebo. Researchers concluded that those patients who took glucosamine experienced less wear and tear on the joints than those who took the placebo. This is especially good news for those who are aspirin sensitive or who cannot take NSAIDs because of allergy or gastrointestinal upset.

• In a study published in the October 1998 issue of the journal *Alternative Medicine Review*, researchers reported that supplementation with 5-hydroxytryptophan (5-HTP) has been shown to decrease symptoms of depression, anxiety, insomnia, and somatic pains in patients with fibromyalgia.

Complement Conventional Therapies—But Don't Close the Door

The studies above represent just a sampling of the multitude of reports now affirming the benefits of complementary and alternative medicine modalities. Yet, in the midst of the appeal and mystery of natural therapies, don't close the door to conventional medicine, for this is where we all turn for the "big stuff." After all, who are you going to call when you have a bacterial infection, chronic illness, or need surgery? Your medical doctor should be at the top of your list for providing an accurate diagnosis and treatment for back pain.

You might wonder if alternative medicine really is a radical new prescription. Here is where we must first take a clue from those in the know—research scientists and some medical doctors who express caution, because most alternative treatments have not passed rigorous clinical trials. No matter what the advertising flyer at the natural food store claims, even the most popular medicinal herbs with pharmaceutical compounds have ingredients that have not been tested and are not scrutinized by the Food and Drug Administration.

The FDA uses a different set of rules to regulate dietary supplements than those covering "conventional" foods and drugs. Under the Dietary Supplement Health and Education Act of 1994 (DSHEA), the dietary supplement manufacturer holds all responsibility for making sure the supplement is safe before it hits the shelf of your supermarket or drug store. If the supplement is found to be unsafe after it is marketed, the FDA is then responsible for taking action. In addition, manufacturers must make sure that the product label's information is truthful and does not make false claims to consumers.

As we learn more about CAM therapies, some may emerge as the best strategies for optimal health, while others may emerge as treatments that could lead to severe side effects. Although a great deal of uncertainty surrounds CAM approaches because they have not been tested as rigorously as prescribed or over-the-counter pharmaceuticals, this does *not* mean they do not work. But as with medications, a CAM treatment that might work for your friend may not be safe for you. I ask that you pay attention to what works for you.

The following CAM therapies represent just some of the "natural" possibilities for back pain self-care. Use this discussion as a beginning and then, as you become empowered to look for safe strategies to end back pain and have optimal health, consult with your health care provider.

A Warning from the American Society of Anesthesiologists

If you are facing upcoming back surgery, take some advice from the American Society of Anesthesiologists (ASA). Avoid the following herbs in the two to three weeks preceding elective surgery due to complications that may occur.

Feverfew	Ginseng
Ginkgo biloba	Kava kava
Garlic	St. John's wort
Ginger	

Calming Pain with Herbal Therapies

By classification, natural supplements contain substances like vitamins, herbs, minerals, and amino acids. A number of these supplements inhibit some of the body's chemicals, called inflammatory cytokines. The cytokines include the interleukins, lymphokines, and cell signal molecules, such as tumor necrosis factor and the interferons, which trigger inflammation and respond to infection. Others block the pain-causing prostaglandins and leukotrienes, chemicals in the body that cause inflammation. There are natural therapies that boost endorphins, the body's natural opioids that relieve pain; other therapies help heal an exhausted immune system and repair damaged tissue.

Because pain is a whole-body problem, influencing your body, mind, and emotions, supplements that increase relaxation and have a calming effect are often useful. Other supplements that help with mild depression or melancholy can also help improve well-being if chronic pain has taken an emotional toll. Natural supplements to promote sounder sleep might be helpful if you awaken frequently because of back pain or the stress of daily living.

How Herbs Are Utilized

Herbs come in various forms including pills, liquids, and bulk (usually for making herbal teas). Some herbs are in capsules made from a whole herb or extract. These are easiest to store and are available at most grocery, drug, or natural food stores. Herbs can also come in liquid form, either as a tincture (made from the whole herb) or as an extract (made from one or more parts of the herb). Herbs that are in a liquid are usually more potent.

Herbs vary in price depending on where they are purchased, how they are processed, and strength. You may find that herbs that are calibrated or measured are also more expensive. Still, these may provide more of the healing element you are trying to ingest. If the herb is not calibrated, it may provide too little—or too much—of the active ingredient.

Variations in Production

Herbal products have a high degree of variation in production. For example, herbs grown in the field may have dissimilar amounts of active constituents because of varying growing conditions. It has been observed with ginseng and valerian that there is a wide deviation in the levels of the herbal product in supplements. Because there is no federal regulation of herbal therapies, products coming out of production facilities may vary greatly in active ingredients.

Always select reliable brands for your dietary supplements. Make sure these brands are stamped USP (United States Pharmacopia, an independent nonprofit organization that sets public quality standards for prescriptions, over-the-counter medications, dietary supplements, and other products). This mark on the product's label signifies that the USP has tested and verified the ingredients, product, and manufacturing process.

Herbs to Ease Back Pain
While many people believe they've never tried a natural dietary supplement, if you've ever gulped a cup of green tea to dull an upset stomach or downed a mug of strong coffee to perk up, you can consider yourself an herbalist—you've used a natural substance to treat a specific symptom. Let's now look at the key herbal therapies that might help ease your back pain:

Boswellia (*Boswellia serrata*), commonly used in Ayurvedic medicine, has been used for centuries as an alternative to aspirin. Though findings on this herb for back pain are limited, a few studies suggest that boswellic acids may possess anti-inflammatory activity at least as potent as common over-the-counter medications such as ibuprofen and aspirin.

What's it for?: Pain reliever.

How it works: It's thought that boswellia inhibits pro-inflammatory mediators in the body, such as leukotrienes. In arthritis patients, boswellia may reduce joint swelling and morning stiffness, help to increase mobility, and reduce pain. This herb has also been found useful in fibromyalgia syndrome and rheumatoid arthritis.

Dosage: Take two capsules of dried herb daily or follow package instructions.

Precautions: May cause slight gastrointestinal effects.

Capsicum (*Capsicum annuum*) includes chili pepper, hot pepper, cayenne, red pepper, Tabasco, paprika, sweet pepper, bell pepper, pimento, and green pepper. Cayenne may be helpful as a pain reliever, particularly when used as rub on the skin (see page 91). Double-blind clinical studies of topical capsaicin creams have shown significant pain relief in patients suffering from the pain of osteoarthritis and rheumatoid arthritis.

What's it for?: Pain reliever.

How it works: Hot peppers contain a substance called capsaicin. When capsaicin is applied regularly to a part of the body, substance P (the neuropeptide that carries pain signals) becomes depleted in that location. Studies show that when substance P is reduced in an area on the body, pain is reduced, too. This also explains why people who consume many hot peppers gradually build up a tolerance.

Dosage: Capsaicin comes in strengths of .025 percent to .075 percent, which is added to a cream base. Follow package directions, and allow two to three weeks to notice a major difference in pain relief.

Precautions: Avoid contact with eyes or open wounds and before using topically; do a skin test for sensitivity. Also, make sure you skin is not irritated before applying, and wash your hands thoroughly after usage. If taken orally in large doses, capsicum may cause stomach upset, vomiting, and diarrhea.

Devil's claw (*Harpagophytum procumbens*) is popular in European countries for the treatment of osteoarthritis, rheumatoid arthritis, and gout. A study published in the German pain journal *Schmerz* found evidence that devil's claw might be helpful for muscle discomfort. This trial evaluated 63 patients with muscular tension or pain in the back, shoulder, and neck. The findings confirmed pain reduction in those who took devil's claw when compared to the placebo group.

What's it for?: Muscle or soft tissue pain. Commission E, the German equivalent of the Food and Drug Administration, has approved the use of devil's claw for degenerative disorders of the locomotor system (arthritis, tendinitis, and back pain).

How it works: Devil's claw contains certain compounds (a group of glycosides called harpagosides) in the root that are thought to reduce the synthesis of inflammatory prostaglandins. This results in a reduction in both pain and inflammation.

Dosage: Available as capsules, dried root in tea, tincture, or extract. Follow package directions.

Precautions: Although devil's claw appears safe, avoid it if you are pregnant, nursing, or taking a blood thinner. Also, some people have reported mild gastrointestinal upset, so avoid devil's claw if you have ulcers.

Feverfew (*Tanacetum parthenium*) was once used to "cure" headaches and "melancholy." It has been used as a folk medicine for menstrual cramps since Greco-Roman times. We know that this herb contains a chemical called tanetin, which may act to reduce inflammation.

What's it for?: Pain reliever; anti-inflammatory properties.

How it works: According to a 1995 study in the chemistry journal *Phytochemistry,* feverfew works similarly to white willow bark in that it reduces prostaglandin levels, therefore decreasing pain and inflammation. Some studies show that extracts of the plant can reduce the body's manufacture of prostaglandins by up to 88 percent.

Dosage: Best taken in leaf powder, tablet or capsule, tea. Take 50 milligrams of dried herb (in capsule) daily or follow the package directions.

Precautions: Feverfew is relatively safe, but anyone with a clotting disorder should consult a physician before taking it. Also, feverfew is not proven safe for pregnant or nursing women and should be avoided by people with pollen allergies.

Ginger (*Zingiber officinale*) has been used throughout history as a pain reliever for arthritis and other related ailments. According to a study published in the November 2001 issue of the journal *Arthritis and Rheumatism*, extracts of this root spice has proved to be as effective as conventional painkillers in a clinical trial. Researchers tested the supplement on 250 people with osteoarthritis. Over a six-week period, some were given a 255-milligram dose of the dietary supplement twice a day. The rest were given a placebo. Two-thirds of those given the ginger pills reported relief from pain.

What's it for?: Pain reliever; anti-inflammatory.

How it works: It is thought that ginger may inhibit substances that cause pain and inflammation.

Dosage: Best taken in dried form (powder, capsule, oil and tea) form. Most studies have used 1 gram daily; follow package instructions or take as needed.

Precautions: No adverse effects have been reported, but those with gallstones are advised not to take this for back pain therapy.

St. John's wort (*Hypericum perforatum*) is the herbal therapy used to lift symptoms of depression. This herb is taken by more than 20 million Germans on a daily basis and has become quite popular in the United States. Minor depression is a common disorder that's underdiagnosed and undertreated. Many people with chronic pain suffer from depression, and it can affect your daily functioning and quality of life. Minor depression is also a serious risk factor for major depression.

What's it for?: Minor depression; anxiety; sleep disorders.

How it works: The active ingredient in St. John's wort, hypericin, appears to affect various neurotransmitters, including serotonin, epinephrine, and dopamine. These are the same chemicals affected by the prescription drug Prozac. St. John's wort may also help to improve sleep because hypericum extract increases the brain's output of melatonin at

---

Signs of Depression

If you have two or more of the following signs of depression, talk to your doctor. There is help available with medications and/or professional counseling.

- Significant weight loss or gain
- Change in appetite (decrease or increase)
- Change in sleep patterns
- Agitation
- Fatigue or loss of energy
- Inappropriate feelings of worthlessness or guilt
- Diminished ability to concentrate
- Indecisiveness
- Recurrent thoughts of suicide or death

---

night. Melatonin is a hormone produced by the body that influences the circadian rhythm and sleep.

Dosage: The accepted dose is 300 milligrams of extract (standardized to 0.3 percent hypericin) three times daily.

Precautions: St. John's wort may cause herb-drug reactions, particularly if taken with SSRI agents. Because St. John's wort can sensitize both the skin and the eyes to sunshine, avoid bright lights if you take this herb.

Nettle (*Urtica dioica*) has been used for years in Germany as a safe treatment for arthritis. In a 2000 study researchers found that stinging nettles not only significantly reduced pain, but also that the level of that pain stayed lower through most of the treatment (see page 75). Nettles contain serotonin and histamine, both neurotransmitters that affect pain perception and transmission at the nerve endings.

What's it for?: Pain reliever; arthritis.

How it works: Nettle contains a variety of natural chemicals that may help to lower pain, swelling, and inflammation. These chemicals also help slow down the actions of many enzymes that trigger inflammation, such as cyclooxygenase and lipooxygenase.

Dosage: Available in tincture, dried leaves and stems, or capsule form. Follow package instructions.

Precautions. Excessive amounts of nettle may cause stomach irritation, constipation, or burning skin. If you are allergic to pollen, avoid nettle.

Turmeric (*Curcuma longa*) has a strong anti-inflammatory compound, curcumin, which is responsible for the yellow color of Indian curry and American mustard. Turmeric is a member of the ginger family and a native of South Asia (probably India). Whole turmeric is more powerful than isolated curcumin.

What's it for?: Anti-inflammatory; pain reliever.

How it works: It is thought that turmeric works similarly to the COX-2 inhibitors (page 194) to decrease inflammation by lowering histamine levels and possibly by increasing production of natural cortisone by the adrenal glands.

Dosage: Labeled as standardized turmeric extract or curcumin. Take 400 to 600 milligrams of turmeric extracts (available in tablets or capsules) three times daily or follow package instructions.

Precautions: May cause gastrointestinal problems. If you are taking anti-coagulant medications, drugs that suppress the immune system, or non-steroidal pain relievers (such as ibuprofen), you should avoid turmeric.

White Willow Bark (*Salix alba*) gives another natural approach to chronic backache. The bark of the white willow tree is a source of salicin and other salicylates, compounds that are similar in structure to aspirin (acetyl salicylic acid).

What's it for?: Anti-inflammatory; analgesic; reduces fever.

Make a Poultice

A poultice is a soft, moist substance spread between layers of gauze or cloth and placed hot or warm onto a body surface to help blood flow and reduce pain. You can make a poultice for back pain by placing the paste of chopped herbs that have been lightly cooked or mashed between layers of cloth. Some people find that a neutral temperature betonite clay poultice has a drawing effect on inflamed tissue, helping to ease the pain and swelling. (Make sure the tissue is not too sensitive to avoid injury.) Add comfrey *(Symphytum officinale)* to the poultice. Comfrey is an anti-inflammatory herb that contains allantoin, which promotes new cell growth. Apply the tepid moist comfrey poultice to the painful site, and allow it to stay in place as long as possible. Repeat several times each day.

Do not ingest comfrey or apply it to gaping wounds, as it is potentially toxic. You can find betonite clay and comfrey at most natural food stores.

How it works: Salicylic acid blocks inflammation, the body's response to injury and illness. In a study published in the *British Journal of Rheumatology,* researchers compared the effectiveness of willow bark (Assalix) with a COX-2 inhibitor (super-aspirin). Both groups reported a decrease in pain. Researchers concluded that there was no significant difference in effectiveness between the two treatments at the doses chosen, but treatment with white willow bark (Assalix) was about 40 percent less expensive.

Dosage: Follow package instructions.

Precautions: White willow bark has the same potential as aspirin to cause gastrointestinal upset and have a blood-thinning effect. Do not take white willow bark along with aspirin or other nonsteroidal anti-inflammatory drug.

Calming Herbs

When any type of chronic pain robs you of sleep, you awaken feeling frazzled and anxious. The following herbs can sufficiently calm you down without causing you to feel "drugged."

Chamomile (*Matricaria recutita*) depresses the central nervous system and also boosts immune power. Chamomile increases relaxation, promotes quality sleep, and can be used to relieve nervousness, upset stomach, and menstrual cramps.

Use chamomile as dried herb in supplements and herbal tea. When making chamomile tea, steep the dried herb or tea bag 5 to 10 minutes in hot water, and drink three or four times a day. If you have ragweed allergies, chamomile may exacerbate your symptoms.

Passionflower (*Passiflora incarnata*) is useful as a sedative, antispasmodic, and mild pain reliever. Passionflower may help to ease insomnia, stress, and anxiety. A study, reported in the July 2001 issue of the *Journal of Clinical Pharmacy and Therapeutics,* concluded that passionflower may decrease pain and reduce muscle spasms—both important for back pain sufferers.

Passionflower is available as tincture, fruit, dried or fresh leaves, or capsules. Follow package directions for dried herb in capsules. Avoid combining passionflower with prescription sedatives, and do not take if pregnant or nursing.

Valerian (*Valeriana officinalis*) has a sedative effect and may be useful in treating insomnia, particularly in helping to reduce the amount of time it takes to fall asleep. Valerian is regarded as a mild tranquilizer and has been deemed safe by the German Commission E for treating sleep disorders brought on by nervous conditions. Unlike prescription or OTC sleep and anxiety medications, valerian is not habit-forming, nor does it produce a hangover-like side effect.

Valerian is available as capsules, tincture, and dried flowers. To ease sleep and combat insomnia, the usual dosage of valerian extract in tablet form is 300 to 900 milligrams taken an hour before bedtime. For stress and anxiety, the recommended dosage is 50 to 100 milligrams taken two to three times each day.

Avoid taking valerian with alcohol, certain antihistamines, muscle relaxants, psychotropic drugs, sedatives, barbiturates, or narcotics.

Over-the-Counter Dietary Supplements

Along with some herbal therapies, a host of over-the-counter dietary supplements may be useful for easing back pain. Here are some of them.

Glucosamine

Glucosamine, a naturally occurring amino sugar found in human joints and connective tissues, is useful in maintaining lubrication in the joints, stimulating cartilage repair chemistry, and slowing the breakdown of cartilage.

In one study, glucosamine was compared to ibuprofen (Advil, Motrin, Nuprin). Initially, pain relief was more rapid with ibuprofen (400 milligrams three times daily) than with glucosamine (500 milligrams three times daily). Yet, after four weeks, symptom relief was equal with the two treatments. This is especially good news for those men and women with back pain from arthritis who are aspirin sensitive or who cannot take NSAIDs because of allergy or gastrointestinal upset.

The supplement form of glucosamine comes from crab, lobster, and shrimp shells. Like other natural dietary supplements, glucosamine is unregulated, so the quality of the product will vary. Glucosamine is available in capsules, tablets, analgesic gel, and liquid form. Do not take if you are allergic to shellfish. If you are pregnant, do not take glucosamine. Glucosamine supplements typically take at least two to four weeks to show any benefits, and they do not always work for everyone.

Chondroitin Sulfate

Chondroitin sulfate is another popular over-the-counter supplement that many people use successfully to ease the symptoms of osteoarthritis, a common cause of back pain. It is thought that chondroitin helps give cartilage strength and resilience. While glucosamine supplements come from shellfish shells, chondroitin supplements are usually made from cow cartilage. Some studies show that chondroitin reduces joint pain significantly, and overall mobility is significantly greater with this supplement. Like glucosamine, chondroitin sulfate appears to be safe and effective for treating arthritis symptoms.

Chondroitin is available in capsules and tablets. Though their long-term safety has never been established, neither glucosamine nor chondroitin appear to have side effects. Researchers still do not know whether you must take the two supplements together or if one is effective taken by alone. There are no studies showing that both supplements are necessary. though manufacturers often mix the two in over-the-counter pain formulas. There is also no research on the safety of combining these supplements with NSAIDs or other newer medications.

SAMe (S-adenosyl-methionine)

SAMe (say "Sammy") is a naturally occurring compound in the body. It has been used in supplement form in Europe for more than twenty years to treat depression and pain. In the United States, doctors have studied SAMe as a treatment for depression, liver disease, and osteoarthritis. SAMe appears to affect some physical processes, including the regulation of hormones and the neurotransmitters serotonin, melatonin, dopamine, and adrenaline—all key regulators of mood.

A new federally funded review of the scientific evidence concludes that SAMe may be as effective as NSAIDs for reducing osteoarthritis pain. Also in this study from the Agency for Healthcare Research and Quality, a federal agency associated with the National Center for Complementary and Alternative Medicine, researchers found that compared to placebo, treatment with SAMe was associated with an improvement of approximately six points in the Hamilton Rating Scale for Depression measured at three weeks. This degree of improvement is statistically as well as clinically significant.

Other preliminary study results behind SAMe are quite promising, since this dietary supplement is thought to have anti-inflammatory, pain-relieving, and tissue-healing properties. At least one large study of SAMe found similar benefit to naproxen, a common nonsteroidal anti-inflammatory drug prescribed to relieve pain and inflammation. Yet, unlike naproxen or other NSAIDs, SAMe has fewer side effects. During clinical trials of SAMe as a treatment for depression, some patients reported marked improvement in their osteoarthritis.

If you are unable to tolerate NSAIDs, you might consider SAMe for chronic back pain. Or you might try SAMe to treat depression. Most studies suggest that SAMe works as well as pharmaceutical antidepressants, yet it works quickly, giving results within one week. Pharmaceutical antidepressants may take as long as four weeks to show benefit.

As with other dietary supplements, follow the package directions. While one 400-milligram pill might help alleviate back pain, it takes as much as 1,600 milligrams daily to get an antidepressant effect, which can be extremely costly.

If you are taking other medication, talk to your doctor before using this supplement. Do not take SAMe with monoamine oxidase inhibitors (MAO inhibitors).

5-Hydroxytryptophan (5-HTP)

5-HTP is typically used to treat mild depression based on the theory that as a precursor to serotonin, a neurotransmitter that has a calming effect, these supplements can increase serotonin levels and influence mood, sleep patterns, and pain control. 5-HTP effectively increases the central nervous system (CNS) synthesis of serotonin. Serotonin levels have been implicated in depression, anxiety, pain sensation, and sleep regulation. In a study published in the October 1998 issue of *Alternative Medicine Review*, researchers reported that supplementation with 5-hydroxytryptophan (5-HTP) was shown to improve symptoms of depression, anxiety, insomnia, and somatic pains in a variety of patients with fibromyalgia.

Follow package instructions with 5-HTP.

Essential Fatty Acids

Essential fatty acids are essential to the immune system because they aid in the production of prostaglandins that counter inflammation. Essential fatty acids are available in oils containing omega-3 (fish oils) and omega-6 (linolenic and gamma-linolenic (GLA), which is found in plant oils such as evening primrose, black currant, and borage.

In the past, the omega-3 fatty acids in fish oil (eicosapentaenoic acid or EPA), as discussed on page 57, were used primarily for rheumatoid arthritis (RA) because RA involves significant inflammation and these fatty acids have anti-inflammatory effects. However, we now know that other types of chronic pain also have inflammation, so EPA may help to reduce this. Also, there are new findings that omega-3 fatty acids in fish oil may alleviate depression. In a study published in the October 2002 issue of the journal *Archives of General Psychiatry*, English researchers found that depressed patients who received a daily dose of 1 gram of an omega-3 fatty acid for twelve weeks experienced a decrease in their symptoms, such as sadness, anxiety, and sleeping problems. More studies are needed to confirm this link, but preliminary findings look positive.

It is important to use EPA in addition to your basic treatment program, not to replace it. When used in doses on the label, no serious side effects are known. Fatty acids enable the body to make more products that tend to decrease the inflammation. Eicosapentaenoic acid is available in capsules without a prescription at your drug store or health food store. It takes twelve to sixteen weeks of EPA therapy before benefits begin.

Vegetarians who want to gain this anti-inflammatory benefit can substitute borage seed oil, black currant oil, flaxseed or flaxseed oil, or evening primrose oil—all said to be rich in gamma linolenic acid (GLA), and they also contain several anticoagulant substances. Flaxseed contains more omega-3 fatty acids than any other plant source. In fact, one gram of flaxseed has twice as much omega-3 as a gram of fish oil. You can also try omega-3 supplements made from algae (such as neuromins). Walnuts have omega-3 fatty acids and can be used as snacks, in salads, or in casseroles and other main dishes.

Caution: There is some concern that internal bleeding may result with large amounts of fish oil capsules, especially when taken with aspirin or nonsteroidal anti-inflammatory drugs.

Super Malic

Malic acid, derived from the food you eat, may play a key role in energy production, especially for those with arthritis and related diseases. In several studies, patients with FMS and other types of arthritis took malic acid. Within 48 hours of supplementation, almost all had improvement in pain. Likewise, upon discontinuation of malic acid for 48 hours, the improvement was lost.

Super Malic, a tablet containing malic acid (200 mg) and magnesium (50 mg), is being studied for treatment of fibromyalgia, which causes deep muscle pain and overall aching. In scientific studies, volunteers with FMS took a fixed dose of Super Malic. While no symptom change was seen in short-term trials, when the dose was increased (up to 6 tablets of

Super Malic, twice a day) and continued for a longer duration of treatment in the open label trial, some reductions in the severity of pain and tenderness were found. (An "open label trial" is one in which the medication is not blinded, meaning the drug being taken is known to both the investigator and the participant.)

Researchers believe that Super Malic is safe and may be helpful in treating arthritis and fibromyalgia, both common causes of back pain. If you try Super Malic with your doctor's consent, consider staying on this therapy for at least two months to receive full benefit.

Bromelain
A natural protein-digesting enzyme found in pineapple (*Iananas comosus*) has an anti-inflammatory effect in the body that may help to ease back pain, arthritis, and fibromyalgia. In uncontrolled studies, bromelain supplements were found to give some relief to rheumatoid arthritis patients, including reduced pain and swelling. Because bromelain dissolves damaged scar tissue and speeds the healing rate of bruises, it is helpful for those who suffer frequently from tendinitis or sports-related injuries such as tennis elbow. Bromelain works in the body by inhibiting the release of certain inflammation-causing chemicals. It is available in tablet or capsule form.

Flavonoids
Flavonoids are chemical compounds widely distributed throughout the plant world. A class of flavonoid derivatives called bioflavonoids also shows important anti-inflammatory properties, including the inhibition of a type of phospholipase involved in the inflammatory response. In a 1999 study published in the journal *Planta Med*, researchers identified a bioflavonoid compound from ginkgo called ginkgetin, which has shown to inhibit the release of arachidonic acid and some of its metabolites. In combination, these data suggest that ginkgetin is a powerful anti-inflammatory substance.

In the study, researchers induced arthritis in laboratory rats, and then treated them with ginkgetin or the drug prednisolone, an oral corticosteroid used to suppress inflammation. Significant reduction in inflammation was achieved with ginkgetin injections, but not with oral administration. Comparison of body and organ weights of rats treated with ginkgetin or prednisolone revealed that while prednisolone decreased spleen and thymus weights, ginkgetin did not. The researchers theorize that the mechanism

---

To Reduce Inflammation and Pain

Limit the intake of omega-6 vegetable oils, such as safflower, sunflower, and corn oil, to no more than one tablespoon per day, as it may increase inflammation. This is especially important if you have any form of inflammation, such as inflamed joints.

---

of ginkgetin's anti-arthritic activity is different from that of prednisolone. A subsequent test also demonstrated that ginkgetin has analgesic activity.

You might try taking 500 milligrams of flavonoids, such as quercetin, three times a day. Quercetin, a water-soluble flavonoid, is available in supplement form at any health food store and is also found in red wine, green tea, onions, apples, and leafy vegetables. Quercetin has potent antioxidant and anti-inflammatory activity, where it can protect cellular structures and blood vessels from the damaging effects of free radicals.

Essential Oils and Rubs

Some herbs work best to relieve pain when they are rubbed into the painful joints or muscles. Here are the most popular herbal salves that I recommend. They can be found at health food stores and most drugstores.

Arnica (*Arnica montana*) is a daisy-like mountain flower that contains *sesquiterpene lactones*, active components that reduce inflammation and decrease pain. In ointment form, arnica tincture acts as an anti-inflammatory

---

Tiger Balm Gives Relief

Tiger Balm, available at most health food stores, is a natural product that gives many of my patients relief from lower back pain. This Asian remedy is filled with potent aromatic herbal extracts—menthol from peppermint, eugenol from cloves, cineole from cajuput (similar to tea tree oil), cinnamon, and camphor. Rub Tiger Balm on the painful site and you might get relief within minutes for mild pain.

---

and analgesic for aches and bruises. Rub arnica tincture into the painful site, but only if your skin is not broken. Arnica may cause a skin rash in some people and should never be taken internally, as it can increase blood pressure and may damage the heart muscle.

Capsicum, an ointment made from the spice in cayenne pepper, is an effective treatment for muscle spasms, tension headaches, osteoarthritis and rheumatoid arthritis, fibromyalgia, back or neck pain. It is also commonly used to relieve pain caused by shingles and surgical scars. Capsaicin, the active ingredient in capsicum, temporarily stimulates the release of substance P in the nerves. This may initially result in pain and burning, but repeated applications deplete substance P, which limits the ability of the nerves to transmit sensations and reduces pain. It's best to use disposable gloves to apply three to four times daily, and if you feel you need to get it off, wipe the area with a dry cloth. If you wet the area, it may burn more. Wash your hands well after use to avoid getting in your eyes, nose, mouth, or private parts.

Capsicum is available as Capsaicin and Zostrix, both are nonprescription drugs and are available at most pharmacies and grocery stores.

Become a CAM Expert

Forty-six-year old Alicia had taken white willow bark, a natural herbal therapy for pain relief (see pages 83–84) for years. As a high school English teacher, she also took gingko biloba and ginseng to increase mental alertness and boost immune function, and valerian to help with insomnia.

Alicia never mentioned taking these natural dietary supplements at her appointment. Yet when I wrote her a new prescription for a stronger NSAID for back pain, I mentioned, "Now don't use this pharmaceutical in conjunction with any other over-the-counter pain reliever or dietary supplement that might have similar properties."

When Alicia heard the word "supplement," her eyes opened wide. "Aren't natural dietary supplements such as herbs considered to be like food? After all, they are natural therapies—not chemicals like drugs."

I've found many patients like Alicia who regularly use natural dietary supplements have very little knowledge of their therapeutic properties, possible drug interactions, or side effects. I explained to Alicia how botanicals often have similar properties to strong pharmaceuticals, depending on their composition. Moreover, just like prescribed medications, herbal therapies have effects—and side effects. They act—and interact—depending on how they are used.

At my request, Alicia wrote down a list of the herbal therapies she was taking at the time. Upon reviewing it, I was particularly concerned with the white willow bark, which has similar action to aspirin, and showed her the precautionary information on white willow. I recommended that she avoid taking this herb in combination with the newly prescribed medication, which I felt would give her better relief for her back pain problem than the natural therapy. I also suggested that in her next office visit, we would reevaluate to see if she still needed the NSAID. If her pain was less, we might consider going back to the daily herbal therapy with white willow.

Just as with prevention and treatment of back pain, you must become your own expert about natural supplements. No, I don't mean you must study herbal medicine, although that's not a bad idea if you have time to learn more about the history and usage of natural therapies! I mean that you need to understand what you are putting into your body and how to discern which complementary and alternative medicines will enhance your health and which might increase your chance of illness.

Talk with your doctor about the benefits and risks of complementary and alternative medicine therapies, and evaluate these factors in terms of your back pain problem and overall health. A good rule of thumb is to make sure the following two criteria are met:

1. The CAM treatment makes you feel better.
2. The CAM treatment does not hurt you in any way.

Potential Herbal-Drug Interactions

Caution! Herbs and medications can have some serious interactions. Check out this chart:

Herb	Drug	Result
Licorice root	Antihypertensives	Hypertension
Garlic, ginkgo biloba	Coumadin, aspirin	Hemorrhage, bleeding
St. John's wort	Antidepressants	Serotonin syndrome
Valerian root	Alcohol, prescription sedatives	Heightens effects

Pain-Free Back: Back to Nature Rx

- Use your Pain-Free Back Diary or PDA to write down the natural dietary supplements you are taking. Be sure to ask your doctor about these supplements to avoid herb-drug interactions.
- Review the herbs that can ease back pain. Consider trying one of these herbs after talking with your doctor. Be sure to read the precautions given and follow any package instructions.
- Make sure the dietary supplements you buy have the USP mark, signifying that the United States Pharmacopia has tested and verified the ingredients, product, and manufacturing process. Although there is no Food and Drug Administration regulation for natural dietary supplements, choosing reputable name-brand items with the USP mark can ensure a better quality of ingredients.
- Instead of ingesting herbs, try those that are compounded in rubs and salves for immediate pain relief. Capsicum (in Capsaicin and Zostrix) is a common household name for many and gives excellent relief after several applications. Follow package directions. Be sure to wash your hands thoroughly, and keep your hands away from your face since capsicum can burn sensitive tissue.
- Even if you have a well-balanced diet, some natural dietary supplements such as flavonoids, enzymes (bromelain), and omega-3 fatty acids found in fish oil and flaxseed might help to decrease inflammation and pain.
- If back pain causes anxiety and sleeplessness, consider trying valerian or SAMe. Both are known to ease anxiety and help you to fall asleep easier. Talk to your doctor if you take other medications to make sure there will be no dangerous interactions.

Back to Basics

Within three months of starting her dental practice, Caroline started having pain that regularly radiated from her lower back to her left hip and thigh. The pain usually started around 2:00 P.M. each workday. As a runner, this active thirty-two-year-old woman thought she had strained her back by pushing herself too hard in a recent race. When stretching, massage, and specific back exercises didn't work to end her pain, Caroline made an appointment to have an evaluation at our clinic.

When I saw Caroline, she was very frustrated, as the back pain was causing her to feel out of control in life and had forced her to stop running, which she loved. As a dentist, she understood inflammation and how to resolve it with moist heat or ice and anti-inflammatory medications. However, none of these self-care measures seemed to be working for her.

After reviewing Caroline's medical history and doing a physical examination, I asked her to show me how she stood while performing her job as a dentist. Caroline stood up and leaned toward an imaginary patient. As she did so, I noticed that she put most of her body weight on her left leg while leaning, which left her body unbalanced. When I mentioned this to Caroline, she said that's how she's stood since dental school; it helps her view her patient's mouth and teeth.

I knew it would not be easy to break this habit. But Caroline was convinced that she could do it. Awareness of the problem is often all you need to take back control and win over back pain.

When I saw Caroline again, she was pleased that her back pain was gone. She said she reminds herself daily to stand correctly, watching her posture and balance. Some days, when standing for prolonged periods during a lengthy procedure, Caroline places one foot on a higher surface (a stool) for a while and then alternates with the other foot to avoid putting pressure on one side of her lower back for too long.

As Caroline realized, often you can make a few basic changes in your lifestyle habits—how you stand, sit, sleep, lift, and carry—to easily resolve chronic back pain. This young woman learned to stop leaning on her left leg while doing procedures on patients at her dental practice. An awareness of the problem was all it took to help her end pain.

While each step in your *Pain-Free Back Program* is equally important, taking control of certain factors can save you a lot of pain and suffering, doctor's appointments, and costly medications. For instance, relearning how to lift heavy objects can save you from a lifetime of horrible pain and even disability. Learning how to stand properly without putting abnormal pressure on the spine may ease the pain you feel. Finding the correct

---

Use Your Pain-Free Back Diary

As you start Step 4 and get "Back to Basics," I want you to become aware of specific activities that result in increased pain or stiffness. For instance, you may notice increased back pain and muscle tension after sitting for several hours at your computer workstation. Or, you might find that lifting your toddler out of his crib puts added pressure on your painful back, making it difficult to stand straight and have good posture. On the other hand, a lengthy automobile ride without any breaks may leave your back aching for days, as can carrying a heavy briefcase or purse.

After you assess your daily living activities. such as getting dressed, meal preparation, and household chores, for problem areas, evaluate your work habits, noting the way you sit, lift, or stand at work that might cause added stress or strain on your back. Write down these concerns in your Pain-Free Back Diary or PDA (page 4).

Just as you did with Steps 1, 2, and 3, as you read this step, make notes in the diary on ways to make basic changes in how you move each day. Talk to your doctor about these basic problem areas and consider meeting with an occupational therapist. A professional can help you make necessary changes in how you move your body and protect your joints, and also give you tips on assistive devices, which can help lighten the load at home and work.

computer or desk chair can help to ease work-related back pain. And learning how to sit properly can keep your back in excellent health.

In this step, let's look at some of the common lifestyle problems that can result in back pain and offer specific suggestions for resolving these problems today.

Computer-Related Back Pain

Lower back pain nagged Judith for months before she came to our clinic for an evaluation. Although this forty-three-year-old magazine editor had a sedentary job, Judith was very active, walking regularly with a group of friends after work, taking a yoga class twice weekly, and doing a regular stretching routine each morning for twenty minutes.

When Judith was sitting at her computer workstation at work, the back pain did not bother her until a few hours into the day. "Almost invariably the pain starts around lunchtime. At first it is a dull ache, then no matter which way I sit on my office chair, the pain intensifies and causes my lower back and right hip to throb."

Judith noticed that after she walked around for a few minutes, the pain lessened. However, at night, the pain would come back when she started working on her home computer, making it difficult to get comfortable when she tried to sleep.

After assessing Judith's symptoms, medical history, and doing a physical examination, it seemed likely that her computer workstation habits and her chair were causing her to sit incorrectly, resulting in poor posture and increased pressure on her back. Over time, poor sitting habits may increase stress on the muscles of the back and even cause damage to spinal structures—while adding to back pain.

Ergonomic Problems Result in Pain and Injury

I suggested to Judith that she identify ergonomic problems at work, and then make specific changes with her computer chair, desk, keyboard, monitor, mouse, and work area. The science of ergonomics has to do with the safety and efficiency of the workplace as it relates to its physical effects on workers. In other words, it refers to fitting the computer workstation to the person, not the person to the workstation. Studies show that in businesses or organizations where workstation furniture is not adjustable or ergonomically correct, it can result in on-the-job pain and stiffness in more than one-third of workers. In particular, in one study published in 2002 researchers evaluated a government office building and found that, as in many workplaces, furniture purchased before the current workstations were were not designed to meet the needs of intensive mouse use for prolonged periods. They found that the chairs often lacked adequate back support, and workers, in an attempt to avoid pain, often assumed positions that were not recommended. Their recommendations? Adjustable furniture and adequate desk and storage space.

Further findings, published in a 2002 issue of the *Annual Review of Biomedical Engineering*, revealed that exposures at work to tasks such as lifting, especially in awkward postures or heavy or repetitive lifting, are directly related to back pain. These researchers found fixed postures and prolonged seating can increase back pain at work, and the prolonged sitting posture and inactivity can lead to more disk degeneration and even disk herniation. It was recommended that better muscle function, avoiding fixed postures, and seats with good lumbar support can help prevent back problems.

Computer-Related Injuries Are Epidemic

It's becoming more apparent that as a nation we've moved into the computer age, but our offices, homes, and schools have not. More than 54 million American households have one or more computers in the home. Add to this huge number the millions of computers used in the workplace, as well as video display terminals (VDTs) used by workers like air traffic controllers and dispatchers, among others. In a study published in the November 2002 issue of *American Journal of Industrial Medicine*, researchers followed 25,000 workers over a period of three years and found that physical symptoms were higher with increasing daily VDT use. Mental and sleep-related symptoms were higher when the VDT was used for more than five hours per day.

While on-the-job injuries used to be the result of heavy lifting or moving large loads, today even sedentary office workers get workplace back pain. Considering the skyrocketing use of computers today, along with flat, light-touch keyboards that permit high-speed typing and pointing devices (the "mouse"), is it any wonder that the number of painful injuries is epidemic?

Certainly, computer technology has revolutionized the way we live and work over the past decade. However, millions of users now suffer with chronic pain problems and disability, including the nagging ache of lower back or hip pain and neck pain. Many computer-related tasks lead

---

The Facts

- There are more than one hundred different types of computer-related injuries.
- Computer-related injuries constitute about one-third of all workplace injuries in lost workdays.
- Computer-related injuries account for one-third of workers' compensation insurance claims.
- According to the Occupational Safety and Health Administration (OSHA), computer-related pain and injuries affect some 1.8 million workers annually.
- Chronic and acute pain costs Americans an estimated $100 billion each year and is the leading cause of medical-related work absenteeism.
- Pain-related problems each year result in more than 50 million lost workdays.

---

to prolonged static (fixed) positioning or malpositioning of the back, neck, arms, and legs, producing rapid fatigue and increasing the risk of chronic pain problems. In addition, with continuous use of the mouse and keyboard, the effect of repetitive motion patterns has led to disorders—some irreversible—in the muscles, tendons, nerves, and joints.

Daily-Living Back Pain

Turn, twist, lift, sit, bend, and reach. As you might have experienced, pain is common in the workplace. The Center for Work and Health at AdvancePCS presented cumulative findings at the Tenth World Congress on Pain, reporting that people bring their pain to work and then do not function efficiently, resulting in tremendous loss of productive work time. This loss of productivity costs businesses billions of dollars annually—money they could save if work environments were people-friendly.

But even the motions of daily living result in excruciating back pain if you aren't careful. My brother-in-law Bob was getting out of bed one Saturday morning, and as he turned around, felt a horrible pain in his lower back. Unable to move, he gently sat down on the bed and realized that every twitch his body made—every small movement—resulted in unbearable back pain.

Take the Posture Test

No matter if you are standing, sitting, or lying in bed sleeping, correct posture is crucial for avoiding back pain. Standing sideways in front of a mirror, drop an imaginary line from your ear to the floor. This line should go through the tip of your shoulder, the middle of your hip, the back of your kneecap and the front of your anklebone. As you assess your posture, pull your abdominal muscles in and notice how your alignment straightens. Do this several times daily as you become more aware of your posture. With the Pain-Free Back Exercise Program, you will strengthen all the key muscles of your body and many posture problems will self-correct.

6 Power Posture Tips

1. Stand tall with your chin parallel to the ground.
2. Pretend you are balancing a book on your head and look forward, not down.
3. Draw your shoulders together as if they are attempting to touch.
4. Pull your stomach toward your spine.
5. Lift up your chest and keep your neck long.
6. Tuck in your pelvis.

Bob knew the rules for ending back pain and began to use a warm shower on his back, three times daily. He slowly began the Pain-Free Back Exercise Program on day two of his painful injury. Bob added a COX-2 nonsteroidal anti-inflammatory drug (see page 194), and went to work on day three. Even though he had some back discomfort, he was able to work a full day and then do his moist heat and exercises that night. Within a week, Bob was back to his usual activities without lifting.

Whether at work, home, or play, you can avoid further back pain problems by making a personal commitment to change the way you sit, stand, walk, lift, and carry on with your daily activities. Let's look at some common types of daily-living back pain and how you can resolve these with self-care methods.

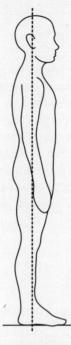

Figure 4.1

Correct posture

SITTING

Problem: Sore tailbone while sitting for long hours at work.

Pain-Free Back Rx: Sitting does put considerable pressure on the spine, which can result in back pain. This puts office workers or those who work at video display terminals at higher risk than other workers for pain and injury. We know that back pain is as common among clerical workers in jobs that require prolonged sitting as it is in workers who do heavy lifting. One revealing study, published in the June 2002 issue of the journal *Spine*, confirmed evidence that sitting slumped can worsen pain for those with back problems. Knowing that the muscles of the lower back and pelvis are important in keeping good body alignment during sitting, researchers concluded that when people slump while sitting, those muscles are less active and therefore give less support. Sitting with legs crossed can also put pressure on the back, resulting in pain (see figure 4.2). Sitting in more erect positions with both feet on the floor or on a stool gives more effective support to the back.

Whether you stand or sit, any static position for lengthy periods can result in pain. Sitting can result in disk degeneration and disk herniation.

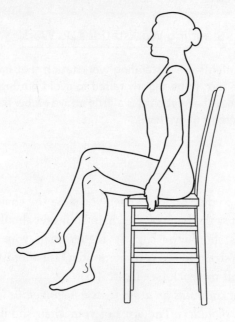

Figure 4.2

Improper sitting posture

For those who drive a car or truck for long periods of time, this sitting posture can also lead to musculoskeletal problems. Be sure to use the following self-care tips to keep your back pain-free!

Use a lumbar disk support. Roll up a thick bath towel and put this
behind your waist when sitting at your desk. Or you can buy a lumbar
disk support at a medical supply store.

Try sitting on a foam cushion. You can protect your tailbone from injury
and pain by sitting on a thick foam cushion. These can be made out of
foam. (Cut a piece of foam the size of the seat of your chair. Cut a 4-inch
circle out of the center to relieve pressure). Or you can buy a ready-made
"doughnut" cushion at most medical supply stores. For a sore tail bone,
protect the point of tenderness at the tip of the coccyx. I have many
patients who carry their cushion with them in a large bag to avoid injury
and to protect that tender point on the tailbone.

Select an ergonomically correct chair with strong back support. Sitting
with no back support increases the force on the spine about 40 percent
more than standing. Leaning forward when you sit causes even higher
forces. A reclined posture with your chair back at a slight angle often

> ## Standing Workstations Do Work
>
> Some of my patients use a standing workstation that has a foot rail. This allows one foot to be slightly raised to avoid putting added pressure on the spine. The keyboard is a little above elbow height and the top of the monitor is at eye level.

works best to keep you pain free. When you sit in the chair, your buttocks should press against the back of the chair. Your feet should be flat on the floor. Your knees should be slightly higher than your hips, and you shouldn't have to strain to see your computer. Use a footstool, if possible, to ease pressure off the back (see figure 4.3).

Make sure your chair has an armrest, as it helps to take some of the strain off your neck and shoulders. The arms of your chair should be able to go

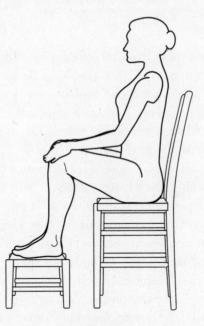

Figure 4.3

Footrest to relieve swayback

under the desk to help prevent the position of sitting and leaning forward. Using an armrest should make you less likely to slouch forward in your chair.

Make sure the height of your desk is comfortable, without requiring you to bend over the work. The arms of your chair should be able to go under the desk to avoid leaning over.

Support your body. If you cannot sit without slouching forward or backward, you need to support yourself with hands and arms or lean against a wall or chair back.

Take a break. Get up and move around for several minutes every half hour. Do some of the stretches listed on page 260 to loosen tight joints, ligaments, muscles, and tendons.

Avoid a fixed sitting posture, and sit "actively." Wiggle around in your chair periodically as you work at a desk for long periods of time. You can rock back and forth and tighten and relax your thigh and pelvic muscles to increase the movement.

Stretch your back. Carefully lean forward to stretch, as shown in figure 4.4. Keep your head down and your neck relaxed, and hold this position for 15 to 30 seconds. Use your hands to push yourself back up in your chair.

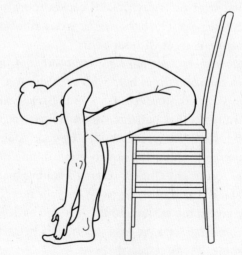

Figure 4.4

Chair stretch

---

5 Tips to End Computer-Related Pain

1. Adjust the computer monitor so that the top of the screen is about 2 inches higher than your eye level. The monitor should be directly in front of you, about an arm's length from your body.
2. Make sure the mouse is within easy reach.
3. Always use a wrist rest with your computer keyboard.
4. Use a document holder to avoid twisting to one side when reading.
5. Don't learn on the chair's armrest when typing, as it puts added pressure on that side of your body.

STANDING

Problem: Back pain from standing.

Pain-Free Back Rx: If your spine is bent over even the slightest bit while standing, the pressure increases on the lower back. The lowest pressure measured on the back is in a standing position with the back straight. You don't need to have perfect posture, but thinking about your back a little can bring great rewards. Here are some specific suggestions:

Keep your back comfortably straight but not overly tense. Standing with your back stooped over or "swaybacked" causes more pressure on the spine and can increase pain. The back exercises described on page 266 can help keep this posture correct without effort.

Wear comfortable shoes that have good support and avoid high heels. Low-heeled shoes can sometimes help with arch support, but more than 1½ inches will misalign the curvature of your back, which can lead to back pain. I recommend that patients choose a lightweight athletic running shoe or proper footwear recommended by your podiatrist.

Vary your standing position. Try not to stand in one position for long periods at a time. You might also try placing a rubber mat in the specific area where you stand if you're going to be on your feet for long periods. The mat helps to give some cushion to the feet and back.

Prop one foot on a box or stool for comfort. This helps to alleviate the pressure on the spine.

Tighten your abdominal muscles as you stand to avoid the "swayback" position. Standing swayback increases pressure on the back and results in pain.

LIFTING

Problem: Back pain during lifting.

Pain-Free Back Rx: The most common cause of lower back pain is using your back muscles in movements or activities you're not used to, such as lifting furniture or doing heavy yard work. It's important to know the facts about lifting to avoid further back injury or pain problems. Did you know that extremely high forces are placed on the lower back when we lift an object? For example, lifting an object weighing 86 pounds (39 kilograms) can cause a force of over 700 pounds on the lower back disks. And this is with *proper* lifting techniques. Heavier weights cause even higher loads on the lower back. When these facts are known, it is surprising that injuries and back pain are not even more common than they are. Since we can't avoid many of these daily tasks, we must become smart in the way we use our backs.

Continue the Pain-Free Back Exercise Program, which will strengthen your back muscles. It makes sense that the stronger and more flexible the back muscles, the more they may be able to tolerate these pressures. Then, proper lifting techniques can help minimize the forces we place on the back.

When lifting, always bend at the knees, not at the waist. Never lift an object by keeping your legs stiff, while bending over it.

Avoid twisting your body. Instead, point your toes in the direction you want to move and pivot in that direction.

Position yourself close to the object you want to lift. Separate your feet (shoulder-width apart) to give yourself a solid base of support. Bend at the knees. Tighten your stomach muscles. Lift with your leg muscles as you stand up.

Use a step stool to reach overhead objects. This can help you avoid unnecessary strain and prevent injury.

Push rather than pull when you must move a heavy object such as furniture or a large box.

Use proper lifting techniques. The National Institute for Occupational Safety and Health (OSHA) has made recommendations to help prevent injuries from lifting. Keep these in mind to help avoid back injuries when lifting. (See page 107).

DAILY-LIVING ASSISTIVE DEVICES

Problem: Performing daily activities without further pain or injury.

Pain-Free Back Rx: For some patients, back pain can turn a seemingly

Assess Job Satisfaction

Could your job be contributing to your back pain? According to some researchers, the answer is *yes*. A report in the February 2003 issue of the *American Journal of Industrial Medicine* concluded that being dissatisfied on the job, or having to work under intense and hectic conditions with many interruptions, can make some workers more likely to feel back pain—more than those who do heavy lifting at work.

In the study, researchers found that when people feel they have little control over their work environment or are dissatisfied with their work, they might feel increased stress. The stress increases tension in their bodies and results in poor posture, which can increase injury. In addition, people who work long hours and have to switch tasks frequently may somehow twist their backs resulting in pain.

The bottom line is to assess your job situation. If you are overwhelmed or feel lack of control, find ways to regain control of your emotional stress using the suggestions in Step 5. On the other hand, if you are unhappy in your position, consider changing to a job that brings you more satisfaction—and less back pain.

easy task such as getting dressed into a virtual nightmare. There are solutions called assistive devices, which can ease the strains of daily activities at home, at work, or at play. Ask an occupational therapist about the latest in daily living assistive devices, or go online and check out the many websites about them (see Resources). Using these specially made tools to take the load off your painful back can eliminate your fear of further injury, falling, or increased back pain:

- A raised toilet seat with grab rails can reduce stress on the lower back and prevent falling.
- A tub grab bar helps to distribute your weight to avoid injuring your back and helps prevent falls.
- A bed pull-up attaches around the bed leg or frame and allows you to pull up and sit in bed without back strain.
- A seat cushion can elevate a chair, making it less stressful on your back to get up and down.
- A firm surface is easier to get up from than a chair with a soft cushion seat.

- A long-handled shoehorn allows you to put on shoes without bending and straining your back.
- Elastic shoelaces allow you to easily slide your foot in and out without having to strain to tie laces.
- A high stool with back support can help alleviate back pain, especially when standing in the kitchen. You can prevent further strain by doing activities at a proper work height.
- A long-handled dust broom and dustpan can keep you from bending during painful flares.
- A trolley on wheels or a wagon can help transport items from one area to another, especially while making meals, putting away food, or working in the garden.

---

8 Ways to Lift without Pain or Injury

1. When you lift an object from the floor, stand close to the object. Start with the center of the weight about 7 to 8 inches from your body. Hold the object close to your body and not at arm's length. Lifting with the arms held out puts higher amounts of stress on the back.
2. Lift with your leg muscles, not your back. This uses the strength of the legs to help take the load off the back muscles.
3. The distance lifted should be no more than 12 to 13 inches for a weight above 86 pounds. If the weight is heavier, the distance lifted should be shorter. If it must be lifted higher, then call for assistance, or use a machine.
4. Try not to lift objects higher than chest level. Lifting above this level can cause much higher stress on the back muscles. If you must reach above your head, use a stool or ladder.
5. Lifting the above weight carefully no more than every five minutes is recommended. If you must lift the weight more often, be sure to follow other guidelines to prevent back injury.
6. Never twist your back when lifting. This puts much more force on the back. If you have to turn, pivot on your feet.
7. Always be sure of your footing. A sudden change in foot placement or a trip can put high force on the back.
8. More force is put on the back when you lift using only one hand, so always use two hands when lifting. Sudden lifting, such as jerking the object, also causes a great increase in force on your back. Try to make lifts smooth and gradual to lower the workload on your back.

HEAVY LIFTING IN THE WORKPLACE

Problem: Back pain with heavy lifting at work.

Pain-Free Back Rx: Consider using a lower back (lumbar) support belt, which are also used by weight lifters. These belts have been found to help decrease the stress on the spine and back muscles when squatting and lifting. These supports also remind you when you forget to use proper lifting techniques.

With continued lifting the muscles of the back and abdomen may become tired and are more likely to be injured with lifting, especially heavy loads. The lifting belt may give added support in these cases and prevent injury after the muscles become more stressed and tired.

If your job demands only occasional lifting, then a back support belt may not be necessary. But if you feel more comfortable with a back support such as a lifting belt, it is acceptable to use. Remember that back supports can't replace proper lifting technique, and no support or lifting belt can replace a regular exercise program to strengthen the muscles of the back. The Pain-Free Back Exercise Program should be continued daily for prevention.

SEX

Problem: Back pain during sex.

Pain-Free Back Rx: Some chronic back pain patients completely give up romantic aspirations for fear of further injury and pain. Being intimate with your spouse or partner is still possible, however, if you take the time

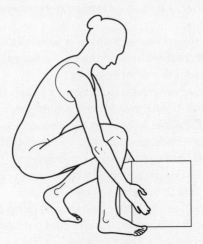

Figure 4. 5

Bend the knees and hips when lifting objects—not the waist.

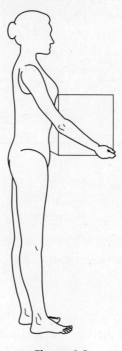

Figure 4.6

Hold objects close to you when lifting them.

to learn some new and comfortable positions for intercourse. Just because you've "always had sex this way," does not mean it's the only way! You'll have to be patient, take it slowly, and find the perfect positions that let you be intimate without causing further pain.

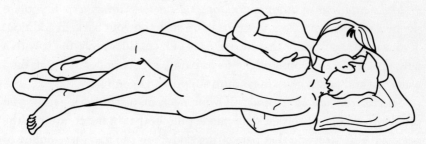

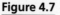

Figure 4.7

For men with back problems, use the side position
with man and woman facing each other.

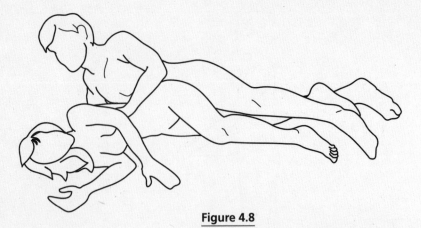

Figure 4.8

For women with back and hip problems, use the side position with the man
behind. Put a pillow between your knees for stabilizing the body.

Your goal is to avoid stress on your back during sexual intercourse. Try
the positions suggested in figures 4.7 and 4.8 and find one that seems
most comfortable. Many back pain sufferers find having their partner on
top or lying on their side (as shown in both figures) is most comfortable.

SLEEP
Problem: Back pain during sleep.

Pain-Free Back Rx: Trying to find a comfortable sleep position with
back pain is not always easy—but it can be done. Getting sound sleep is
important to feel alert and productive the next day. However, when
nights of tossing and turning rob you of precious sleep, it is time to do
some homework. Here are some suggestions:

Make sure your mattress is firm for good support during sleep. If you are
sleeping on a soft mattress, this puts extra stress on your back. In addition,
if your mattress is more than three years old, consider replacing it with a
new firm mattress. Some of my back pain patients prefer sleeping on a
waterbed and find it gives maximum support and comfort.

Select a comfortable position. If your neck or upper back causes you
problems, try one of the specially made pillows that fit the contour of the
neck and ease stress on that part of the body. You can find these online or
at any medical supply store.

*If you have arthritis in the spine, try to sleep on your stomach for at least a
brief period each night.* This can help to prevent posture problems, particu-

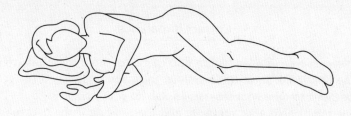

Figure 4.9

Lie on side with knees bent to flatten the back.

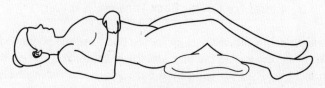

Figure 4.10

Lying on back is correct if knees are supported.

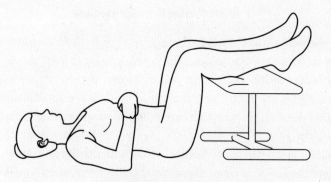

Figure 4.11

The 90/90 rest position can alleviate lower back pain.

larly the "stooped over" appearance that is a common problem in many types of spinal arthritis, especially ankylosing spondylitis (see page 180).

Continue your Pain-Free Back Exercise Program (Step 1) to increase muscle strength. Your posture will also improve without your thinking about it. Along with exercise, the above suggestions to avoid unnecessary forces on the back during sleep will improve the results even further.

Correct Imbalance

Sometimes having a leg length discrepancy of more than 1.25 cm can cause back pain. Since this is only ½ inch, you might try a corrective shoe insert to raise your shorter leg. Talk to your podiatrist to see if an insert might help your problem, and then decide if the back pain is improved.

Relief for Lower Back Tension and Pain

To release a painful lower back or locked back, use the 90/90 rest position to take pressure off the hips and lower spine. You can do this, as shown in figure 4.11, by lying on a flat surface and flexing both hips and knees to 90 degrees. Use a coffee table, piano bench, or couch to rest the legs.

7 Joint Protection Strategies

One of the best things you can do to save your back from more pain and injury is to protect your joints, which reduces local joint stress and preserves joint integrity. Each time you twist or turn the wrong way or lift incorrectly, you are increasing the stress on delicate muscles and joints. Over time, these strains can increase inflammation and degeneration. Prevention is the key!

Evaluate your habits at home, work, and during exercise or recreational sports. Do you overextend your body even when you feel tired? Do you hurry to get some jobs done yet at the risk of possible injury? Make sure you understand and following these 7 joint-saving strategies to prevent back pain from happening again.

1. *Respect pain.* Pain is your body's warning signal that it is time to stop, slow down, or readjust how you are performing a task. When you feel pain, stop what you're doing. Assess the pain before you continue the exercise or activity. Listen to your body and don't ignore the signals it gives you.

2. *Balance work and rest.* You know the saying, "Even strong horses have to rest." Well, I tell patients that all work and no rest sets them up for acute back pain. It's true. Your body needs to rest between exertions and exercises in order for stressed muscles to heal and rejuvenate. Make sure you allow this time.

3. *Maintain strength and range of motion.* Muscles and joints must be stretched daily to maintain flexibility. When you are flexible, you bend and move easier and the risk of back pain is less. Anyone can become flexible by starting the Pain-Free Back Exercise Program (Step 1). Make sure you continue this program after your back pain is gone to keep your back strong and injury-free.

4. *Reduce musculoskeletal effort.* Be sure you choose the most efficient way to use your back for every heavy task. For example, lift objects with your legs, not your back, as shown in figure 4.5. Instead of bending your back during the lift, keep your back erect as there is less force transmitted to the spine. In addition, lift holding objects close to the body, not with arms extended.

5. *Avoid positions that induce deformity.* Sleeping for hours on your side with your spine bent and knees flexed in a fetal position. Sleeping for hours with your knees flexed on a pillow. Sitting in a chair for prolonged times in a slumped position or in a slumped position leaning forward. Instead, try walking with your back upright in posture as in figure 4.1. This produces less force on your spine than sitting.

6. *Use stronger, larger joints whenever possible.* When lifting, use your leg muscles to carry the load instead of your back muscles. Bend at your knees and keep your back straight. Use your large thigh muscles to give you strength as you lift the object with both arms instead of one hand.

7. *Avoid staying in one position for too long.* When sitting for long periods, shift around in your seat. Or get up and walk around every 15 minutes to avoid putting abnormal pressure on the spine. Break up tasks such as standing for long periods by walking around, bending and stretching, or propping your foot on a stool to relieve strain on the back.

Fall-Proof Your Home

Falling is a major reason many people live with chronic back pain. With the increase in age, the tendency to fall increases too, and women tend to fall more often than men. I've treated men and women who fell and injured their backs after tripping on objects such as lawn furniture or kids' toys, slipping in the bathroom because of no safety equipment, and falling over a decorative bedside rug when it bunched up and the room was too dark to see it. Several of my patients injured their backs when running down stairs with sandals or socks on. Imagine how slippery—and painful—that must have been!

The stories are endless about how people fall, but for the most part this type of injury can be prevented with some proactive measures taken to ensure personal safety at home. Review the following suggestions and make sure your home is safe—not only for you, but also for your family and guests who come to visit.

1. *Check the lighting.* Poor visibility is the cause of many falls. Studies show that as we age, we need *two to three times* as much illumination as young adults. Make sure your home is well lit throughout, including hallways and outside paths. Replace burned-out bulbs and have nightlights on in hallways, bathrooms, and bedrooms at night to prevent injuries.

2. *Make sure your walkways are safe.* Check them daily for any items that could obstruct the path and cause a fall. Pick up any debris, including shoes, telephone and lamp cords, and children's toys, or any other objects that impede the pathway. Make sure your outside path is free from leaves, puddles of standing water, wet snow, or ice. Also, coil all garden hoses and store near the house and away from the entrance. Devices are available at your garden store to hold the hoses safely.

3. *Secure all carpeting.* If you have throw rugs, make sure they have a rubber mat that adheres to the bottom of the rug and to the floor, so they don't bunch up or slide. Clean under throw rugs regularly, since dirt or sand under the rugs will cause them to slide when walked on. Reglue vinyl flooring if it is coming loose, and have any loose floor tiles repaired.

4. *Make sure all electrical cords are out of sight.* Keep lamp cords and other electrical wires and cords behind the furniture so they are not a falling hazard.

5. *Wear good support shoes that grip.* Slippers, socks, women's mules or clogs, and sandals, among others, are the common reasons why many people fall at home. If you have sturdy shoes on, your chance of falling is reduced.

6. *Add nonslip strips, bath mats, and grab bars in the bathroom.* Always sit on the tub and slowly lift your legs in the water to avoid slipping while standing. Make sure your feet are securely grounded on the floor as you get out of the bath or shower, and wipe up water splashes immediately.

7. *Use a nonskid stool with a back in the bathtub for moist heat treatments.* You might consider a water-resistant and height-adjustable "bathbench" or chair. This bench lets you sit at a normal height in the bathtub while bathing and is safe for moist heat applications.

8. *Make sure your bedspread fits tightly and does not slip off the bed.* The dust ruffle should be off the floor instead of touching it. If you have wood floors, do not use a glossy cleaner that adds shine to avoid creating a slippery surface. Remove any throw rugs next to your bed as these can bunch up or slip.

9. *Make sure all stairways and steps have secure railings.* Put colored tape on the top and bottom step to remind you to proceed with caution. Never go up or down stairs without sturdy shoes on.

10. *Keep small pets on leashes when company comes.* This is especially important if older adults are visiting in the home, since they may not see the animal in their path.

11. *Be careful with medications.* If you take medications that cause you to feel drowsy, take extra precautions when you walk or move around to avoid falling. Talk to your doctor or pharmacist if medications make you feel drowsy, dizzy, or unsteady. Taking multiple medications can increase the risk of falls, especially in older adults.

12. *Watch alcohol consumption.* Even a small amount can affect your coordination and reaction time. Falls are much more common in those who drink alcohol, especially in excess.

13. *Stay alert.* Depression, decreased memory or concentration, and other cognitive impairments also increase the risk of falls. Certain conditions like decreased vision, arthritis, muscle weakness, multiple medications, or other illnesses put an elderly person at risk of falls. Awareness of the higher risk can help increase care to prevent falls.

14. *Fall-proof yourself!* Regular exercise with the Pain-Free Back Exercise Program will help you maintain the strength and coordination necessary to avoid falls and also keep bones strong to prevent injuries when you do fall. Tai chi (discussed on page 27) has been shown to improve balance and flexibility, both necessary for reducing risk of falling. Studies show that tai chi can actually reduce the risk of falling, especially in older people.

Gardening Tips

Gardening is an active pastime for many people. Not only does this hobby let you get outdoors and enjoy nature, but you also benefit from the gardening "moves"—bending, pulling, pushing, digging, raking, sweeping, and more. Gardening increases flexibility, strength, and stamina, which are all important for keeping the back healthy and strong.

The problem with gardening and back pain is that many people are afraid to tackle a garden after a bout of acute back pain. Chronic back pain sufferers may lock the gardening shed indefinitely for fear they'll reinjure their backs. An interesting Gallup poll (2000) of more than 2,000 adults found that nearly 42 percent had suffered from back pain

---

Stop Smoking

Smoking increases the risk of osteoporosis, which results in painful fractures. Nicotine in cigarettes interferes with the supply of nutrients to the disks, making them more susceptible to injury.

5 Basics to End Back Pain Today

1. Check for pressure placed on the pelvic bones by a wallet, tight belt, or constricting jeans that can squeeze nerves in the pelvis or groin.
2. Don't carry a heavy purse.
3. Wheel your belongings instead of using a briefcase or backpack.
4. If you do use a backpack, make sure you balance the weight on both shoulders instead of slinging it on one shoulder, which can result in back pain.
5. Try a fanny pack instead of a purse for long day trips.

and nearly half of these adults (about 47 percent) said their back problems were a result of working in the garden.

If gardening is your passion, but you've given it up because of back pain, consider the following tips to continue enjoying your fresh flowers, fruits, and vegetables without strain or further injury to the back:

- Plant low-maintenance shrubs and perennials.
- Plant from a kneeling position. Use "kneeler seats" with handles or mats, not low seats.
- Help take the strain off your back by using long-handled tools such as rakes, hoes, and shovels.
- Follow the rules for lifting on page 107 when you must lift a large plant, soil, fertilizer, or mulch.
- Stop periodically during your gardening time to stretch your body. One good stretch is to bend backwards while standing. Put your hands in the small of your back (by your waist) and slowly bend backwards to counteract the forward bend you've been doing. Do this stretch several times and then resume your gardening.
- Get organized before you start. Gather your gardening supplies and keep them by your side as you dig, plant, or weed. This will help you to avoid back pain or strain from lifting heavy objects.
- Use planters to avoid bending for long periods. Many of my patients use the Earthbox (www.earthbox.com). This box looks like a planting tub but is built higher, so you don't have to lean over to plant and cultivate the garden. With the Earthbox, you never have to

weed, and it's self-watering. You can also use container gardening or raised beds to avoid unnecessary stooping or bending. This type of gardening will allow you to enjoy nature and your favorite plants without strain or pain.

- Use a gardening cart or wheelbarrow to move plants, potting soil, rocks, and other gardening materials. It's easier to move several items by pushing a wheelbarrow than to lift each item and move it individually. Try a lightweight plastic cart that is easy to move when necessary.

Pain-Free Back Basics Rx

- Make sure your computer chair is ergonomically correct.
- Check the position of your computer monitor to avoid leaning forward, which can cause poor posture and back strain.
- Check how you sit in your computer or desk chair. Follow the self-care suggestions to make sure you are doing all you can to keep back pain at bay.
- Evaluate your posture to consciously keep it straight.
- When standing for prolonged periods, place one foot on a higher surface (stool or phone book) for a few minutes and then alternate.
- Relearn how to lift correctly. Make sure you abide by these suggestions to avoid pulling or straining your back.
- Always bend at the knees, not at the waist.
- Evaluate your mattress and make sure it is firm, giving your back full support at night.
- Protect your joints to prevent further injury.
- Fall-proof your home to avoid further injury and pain.
- Consider assistive devices and see if these might help you to stay pain-free in daily activities.

The Pain-Free Back
Relaxation Therapies

Just when you think you can't handle any more interruptions in life, your back gives out on you.

"Why now?" patients ask. "I don't have time to deal with back pain with all my other responsibilities."

I've seen this happen repeatedly. Patients come in with excruciating back pain and need pain relief—fast. This flare-up might coincide with other major life events such as a child going away to college, financial problems, re-careering, or buying a new home. Sometimes, a physical factor, such as lifting or sitting for too long, combines with stress and results in a painful back. Anxiety and tension signal your body to feel everything—including back pain—more acutely.

No matter when it happens, back pain can increase your stress tremendously, and stress can accentuate your pain. In fact, pain and stress have similar effects on the body as muscles tense, breathing gets fast and shallow, and heart rate and blood pressure increase.

Tom's first encounter with back pain happened when he was thirty-three and had started a management trainee program with a Fortune 500 company. He thought nothing of the nagging backache at the time; he was young and the pain resolved itself in a few days without treatment. Nevertheless, when his back pain came back again during the Christmas holidays, and then again, right before summer vacation, Tom's concern increased.

When I examined Tom, he was thirty-five and appeared to be a healthy young man in good physical condition. A former baseball player during college days, Tom had his share of injuries, but they didn't seem to be related to the back pain. So, Tom and I talked about his personal life. Tom said that he and his wife were expecting their third child and were renovating an older home they had purchased the previous year. He had just been promoted to district manager with his company, which meant he had to travel several days each week, leaving his wife home alone with the children.

"I feel like my life is an interminable race," Tom said. "The problem is that in the midst of running faster and harder each day to meet with my business clients, take care of my family's needs, or redo the plumbing in my home, I feel as if I can never reach the finish line. That's about the same time my back pain flares, which immobilizes me."

Just hearing about Tom's busy life made me feel a bit stressed! I explained to him that stress doesn't cause back pain, but the resulting anxiety can cause painful muscle tension and spasms. I also suggested that his back pain might be a warning sign that he was not responding to life's stressors in a healthy way, and he could manage most stressful situations by altering his response. In other words, instead of feeling stressed out as all the demands of life pile up—new job, new baby, new home—Tom needed to find some viable way to reduce his pent-up anxiety and tension before his physical health was negatively affected.

Take Notes in your Pain-Free Back Diary

Do you find that your back pain correlates with times of great stress? Do the muscles in your lower back seem tense at the end of the workday? These are important signs to notice as you learn to relax *before* you suffer the symptoms of stress-related back pain. As you read Step 5, try to identify stressors in your life. Write down these specific events or situations in your Pain-Free Back Diary (see page 4). If you are feeling more anxious than usual, try to figure out if there is a reason, and record it. Also, record how you feel—your specific stress-response symptoms (rapid heart rate, insomnia, asthma, back pain) and emotional state (anger, irritability, depression). In order to maintain your mental balance through stressful events and harried times, you must give yourself opportunities for relaxation. Learn to remove yourself from the stressor and elicit the relaxation response using the mind-body modalities discussed in this step. As you learn to respond differently to the stressors in your life, you'll find that your back pain will decrease, too.

Understanding Stress

Stress describes the many demands—physical, mental, emotional, or chemical—you experience each day. It includes the stressful situation (stressor) and the symptoms you experience under stress (stress response). Stress can be negative (distress) or positive (eustress). (Although getting married, having a baby, and buying a new home are exciting events, they also create stress in your life!)

Science now recognizes that the mind and body are interconnected to an extent far surpassing previous assumptions and that physical health and emotional well-being are closely linked. We now know that daily stress, such as a constantly ringing phone or hearing the sound of "You've got mail!" repeatedly, can lead to emotional turmoil that can shock an immune system into a downward spiral, resulting in chronic or serious illness—and yes, back pain. Is it any wonder that an estimated 90 percent of all doctor visits to are due to stress-related problems? Nearly one-half of all adults suffer adverse effects from stress, and approximately one million Americans miss work due to stress-related complaints.

For those with back pain, stress is nothing new. You may experience stressors such as limitations in activities at home and in the workplace, financial problems because of loss of income and health care costs, and problems with relationships. Some patients find they are more irritable when back pain flares and they prefer to be alone, avoiding social contact. Others say their anger level increases and they become full of self-pity. Then there are those patients who ignore healthy habits when they are under great stress. They stop exercising, eat and drink too much, smoke cigarettes, and become sedentary, among other behaviors.

Many studies show the high frequencies of sleep disturbances with back pain, possibly because of painful joints and surrounding soft tissues. Fifty-three-year-old Holt said that he went without solid sleep for days when he fell on his back at work and fractured a vertebra. "Every position I tried seemed to put more pressure on my lower back," he said. "Finally, I gave up and sat in my reclining chair with a moist heating pad on my back, watched old movies and dozed all night."

No matter what emotional stress you face with back pain, there are answers. This step of the *Pain-Free Back Program* will give you easy ways to de-stress before you become overwhelmed and out of control.

Signs and Symptoms of Stress

Anger	Inability to concentrate
Anxiety	Insomnia
Apathy	Irregular menstrual periods
Back pain	Loss of sexual function
Chest pain or tightness	Loss of sexual desire
Colitis	Mood swings
Depression	Neck pain
Headaches	No energy
Heart palpitations	Rapid pulse
Hives	Rashes
Irritable bowel syndrome (IBS)	Short temper
Impotence	Short-term memory loss
Inability to relax	Weight gain or loss

Indirect Effects of Stress on Your Back

Chronic stress can result in unhealthy habits such as the following, which increase your risk of back pain:

Smoking
Sedentary lifestyle
Overuse of alcohol
Poor eating habits
Social isolation

Rate Your Stress: Acute or Chronic

If you have an acute, stressful emergency that lasts for only a short time, no permanent physical damage is usually done. (In biological terms, a short time would be a few hours, perhaps even a couple of days.) Your heart rate and blood pressure increase as adrenaline floods your body; the heart beats faster and the blood flow to muscles and intestines changes. This adrenaline "rush" prepares you to fight the wild beasts, as in cave days (life's problems). We have a built-in mechanism called the "fight or flight" response that causes a profound set of involuntary physiological changes that allows us to handle acute stressful events. This response is controlled by the hypothalamus in the brain. When we face fear—or even recall a stressful or frightening event from the past—the resulting hormonal changes supercharge our bodies to a state of high arousal to prepare us for action.

However, when stress happens for days or weeks, it is called chronic stress. Chronic stress occurs when we face stressors over a period of time. If we do not have a healthy way of responding to stress or counterbalancing the fight-or-flight response, the constant exposure to stress hormones eventually cause our body to become overloaded, which can lead to physical and psychological problems. Chronic stress can cause anxiety, insomnia, depression, gastrointestinal problems, and dependency on drugs and alcohol.

How Stress Affects Your Health

Not only is stress uncomfortable, causing you to feel nervous or have disturbed sleep, it is also linked to the following illnesses:

Allergies, asthma, and hay fever
Arthritis
Back pain
Cancer
Chronic pain
Heart disease
High blood pressure

Migraine headaches
Temporomandibular joint
   syndrome (TMJ)
Tension headaches
Stroke
Ulcers

Stress Increases Abdominal Fat

Abdominal fat or an increase in waist size can increase your back pain (see pages 40–41). Numerous studies show that the high cortisol secretion associated with chronic stress is associated with abdominal fat. A revealing study in the September 2000 *Psychosomatic Medicine* found that, particularly in women, stress-induced cortisol secretion may contribute to abdominal fat (high waist-to-hip ratio), which increases the risk of chronic and serious illness.

Finding Your Inner Circle of Quiet

"I get high anxiety just lying in bed thinking about what I have to do before the opening day of school," Karin, a principal at a local high school, said. "And then my lower back begins to ache for days. I get low back pain again before the Christmas holidays when there are so many school activities happening, and again during exam week. I always have a backache the last week of school."

I'll never forget Karin. This forty-five-year old mother of four teenagers was an excellent manager, and it showed in her many accomplishments. However, when she couldn't understand why she invariably got back pain without "any reason," I helped her target the culprit—stress. In addition, job stress is the leading source of stress for adult Americans, so Karin certainly had a lot of company.

In order to end her recurring problem with back pain, Karin needed to get in control of how she emotionally responded to her work and family stress. I explained to her that when we have calming thoughts, we tend to have a similar emotional response and comparable physiological effect— we feel in control of our life and our health. When we have angry or anxious thoughts, we are more emotionally aroused. Consequently, when we harbor nervous tension inside, it can result in painful back spasms.

Karin had to find a quiet place each day where she could be alone with her innermost thoughts and feelings. I recommended that she take time out each morning before students arrived on campus and meditate in her office for fifteen minutes. This would give her a sense of calm before work stressors became overwhelming. Then, once she got home from school, Karin might go to her bedroom and do some relaxation exercises or listen to soft music before the busyness of raising a large family became too much for her to handle.

Karin found these suggestions helpful. She realized that the more she gained control of her personal response to stress, the more productive and efficient she was at school and the more congenial was her relationship to her family. Over a few weeks, her back pain subsided, and now she only has occasional flare-ups when she lifts or sits incorrectly or when she neglects to take time for herself.

7 Pain-Free Back Mind-Body De-stressors

Let the following Pain-Free Back suggestions help you to unwind, de-stress, and get back in control of your emotional state.

1. *Identify and eliminate your stressors.* What's causing added stress in your life? Other than your back pain, is your job increasing your stress level? Is it a friend or other person? What about driving to work each day on the crowded interstate? While identifying stressors may be easy, eliminating them is a challenge. Avoiding stressful situations such as heavy traffic, loud noises, ringing phones, large crowds, the neighbor's barking dog, long lines at the grocery store, or even certain incorrigible people is often the best way to handle stress overload—before it results in a physical symptoms (back pain). If you are stuck in traffic or long lines at the grocery store, take ten slow deep breaths at these tense times to stay calm and relaxed. (See how to elicit the relaxation response with deep abdominal breathing on page 134.)

2. *Talk it out.* Talk to a friend, family member, or mental health counselor if your stress level is too high. Getting your feelings out without being judged is crucial to good mental health. Fifty-seven-year old Martha had suffered with degenerative disk disease for more than five years. Though exercising, moist heat applications, and medications helped a lot, she still had a nagging pain in her back when she overdid it.

"It was to the point where I felt hopeless," Martha said. "A friend suggested that I see a professional counselor. After a few sessions, I realized that simply talking openly about my frustrations virtually changed the way I felt. For years, I bottled up all my feelings and didn't want others to know how angry or frightened I was at times. But after undergoing mental health counseling, I'm like a new person. I am more honest with my feelings, and if my back is hurting, I admit it to family and friends instead of trying to hide it."

Psychological counseling can help you to develop coping skills so life's stressors along with back pain do not overwhelm you. Some viable options include:

- Individual counseling—a one-on-one session with a therapist in which your problem areas are addressed. These sessions may include specific help with alleviating depression, anxiety, or stress, along with other personal problems.

- Family counseling—family members gather with a therapist to learn how to understand and accept your problems and the possible impact these may have on your family's lifestyle. If your chronic back pain makes it difficult to participate in family activities and chores, a counselor can help your family to understand what you face during painful flare-ups.
- Group counseling—sessions led by trained therapists that allow for the sharing of feelings with others suffering from stress, as well as the development of effective coping strategies. The exchange of ideas at group sessions is often the most productive way to revamp your thought processes.
- If you are feeling angry, frightened, or depressed, talk to your doctor and see if medication or professional counseling might be helpful.

3. *Take time out.* Before you reach your breaking point from life's unending stressors, take a time-out for solitude. Being alone does not mean feeling lonely, for we can feel lonely in the midst of a crowd or even sitting with our family and friends. Being alone can help you find meaning in your life. Take time to nurture yourself, away from the cares and responsibilities of the world, and find time for inner strength and mind, body, and spiritual healing.

A host of studies show that people who focus on their spiritual side are better able to handle the pain and limitations of chronic illnesses. At the American Geriatric Society's annual meeting in May 2002, researchers from Johns Hopkins reported on 77 patients aged thirty or older who had suffered from rheumatoid arthritis for at least two years. Rheumatoid arthritis is an inflammatory disease that causes severe pain, swelling, and stiffness in many joints. In the study, researchers defined spirituality as "the capacity of an individual to stand outside of his/her immediate sense of time and place and to view life from a larger, more detached perspective." Although being spiritual did not reduce the effects of the rheumatoid arthritis or lessen joint pain, the spiritual patients were much happier and felt better about their overall health and well-being.

By taking time out daily to focus on relaxation techniques such as meditation, deep abdominal breathing, music therapy, or even yoga, you can boost this inner sense of purpose in your life. Volunteering to help others is yet another way to feel more connected spiritually as you stop dwelling on your pain and focus on giving to others.

4. *Set limits.* Never hesitate to say no before you are overextended with too many commitments. Especially if you are balancing career, children, and other commitments, you should not feel guilty about prioritizing what is humanly possible. Take time weekly to evaluate your commitments and only do those that are most important, saying no to the remaining tasks. Saying no, when appropriate, can bring your stress to a manageable level and give you some control over your life. When patients have a hard time saying no, I tell them to write down several polite ways to say no to a friend. For example:

- "No, I am so overcommitted as it is."
- "No, I simply don't feel I can do that right now."
- "While I feel honored that you've asked me to do this, I promised myself not to make another commitment right now."
- "I'd love to help you, but I cannot stand that long because it bothers my lower back." (Be honest about your back problem—no excuses!)

When you are able to follow through with your commitments, you can live your life without undue pressure and stress.

5. *Strengthen your social support.* Connections to a partner, family, and friends, or a support group have been shown to improve mood and ability to cope and can even strengthen your immune system. Most people who are able to cope with stress have strong social support networks with family, friends, and even pets.

Some important types of support include:

- *Emotional support.* This is someone you trust with your most intimate thoughts, anxieties, and fears, and who trusts you.
- *Social support.* This is someone you enjoy being with, who helps you cope with disappointments, and who celebrates your joys.
- *Informational support.* Someone you can ask for advice on major decisions.
- *Practical support.* Someone who will help you out in a pinch (neighbors, a relative, or co-workers).

Who can you turn to for emotional, social, informational, and practical support? Try to identify these key people in your life and work to nurture these much-needed relationships. If you are having trouble thinking of people in any one of these areas, please realize that this is an important task you have to do—reach out to broaden your personal relationships.

6. *Consider joining a support group.* This form of mind-body therapy is geared toward the unique needs of its members, providing both emotional

---

Consider Psychotherapy

Psychotherapy is an effective behavioral treatment that allows you to change your own biology without invasive treatment or medications. Especially for those of you who obsess with negative thoughts, are highly anxious, or even depressed about their situation in life, psychotherapy lets you identify then verbalize inner conflicts as you learn positive coping skills.

In a study published in the July 2002 issue of the *Journal of Rheumatology,* researchers reported that behavioral therapy boosts functioning in patients with fibromyalgia. Fibromyalgia causes chronic, deep muscle pain, along with painful trigger points throughout the body, including the spine. Patients with this syndrome also have depression, sleep disorders, ongoing fatigue, and a host of other physical problems.

In this particular study, 145 fibromyalgia patients were given standard treatment, including pain relievers, antidepressants, and exercise instructions. Half of these patients were also enrolled in six sessions of cognitive behavioral therapy with an experienced mental health counselor which aimed at teaching patients skills to improve their physical functioning. The patients were taught relaxation techniques, as well as how to remove negative thinking from their thought process.

After one year, the researchers found that 25 percent of fibromyalgia patients who underwent behavioral therapy reported a significant improvement in physical functioning after the treatment. This improvement was seen in only 12 percent of fibromyalgia patients who did not receive it.

Studies like this one underscore the great importance of a multifaceted program like *The Pain-Free Back* to beat back pain and other pain problems. The program should include exercise, lifestyle changes, and medications, as well as relaxation therapies and behavioral counseling to target areas that might be contributing to your stress and daily pain.

support and education in dealing with illness or life's stressors. While support groups are not psychotherapy groups, they can give you a safe and accepting place to vent frustrations, share personal problems, and receive encouragement from others. The assurance is given that "someone else knows what I am going through," as people share their personal struggles. As discussed above, having a close bond with others is most necessary to revamp your thought processes and manage your back pain.

7. *Laugh!* No matter how bleak situations look, life goes on. Learn to laugh more and worry less. During stressful times, rent some funny videos and watch them instead of the nightly news. You'll sleep better after a good laugh, and your pain may be reduced as well.

An interesting study found that even looking forward to laughter—or anticipating fun—can help boost the immune system and reduce stress. In this Canadian study, presented at the March 2003 meeting of the Society for Neuroscience, researchers tested sixteen men who were all in agreement that a specific videotape was humorous. Half of these men were told three days in advance that they'd watch this video. This group began to experience biological changes immediately. When the men actually watched the video, levels of the stress hormone cortisol declined by 39 percent. Epinephrine (adrenaline) also fell by a startling 70 percent and endorphin levels (the feel-good hormone) rose 27 percent. Human growth hormone levels climbed 87 percent.

Laugh—and look forward to having fun in the midst of your daily living!

Get Connected

If the thought of making time for friends adds to your stress level, consider getting a pet. Countless papers have been published in the area of animal-human bonding that reveal the health benefits of social support. Even having a plant can be beneficial to your health, since it gives you a sense of purpose and connectedness. This was demonstrated in a Yale University study by Dr. Judy Rodin, who found that when nursing home patients were given a plant to take care of and were told that the nursing home staff was there as a resource, these patients had a 50 percent lower mortality rate than patients who were told they would be completely cared for by the staff.

Mind-Body Therapies You Can Learn at Home

Most of our stress and emotional distress comes from deep inside our mind—how we think and approach life's situations and interruptions. Moreover, these stressful thoughts are usually negative and distorted, since they come from our perceptions, not necessarily what is real. Moreover, we all have the tendency to make situations appear a lot worse than they really are. This is called *awfulizing* (for example, your doctor's office calls and leaves a message on your voice mail that your test results are back, and you immediately think, "Oh, no! The test was positive."). Using mind-body therapies effectively each day will help you stop thinking of worst-case scenarios and let you focus positively on resolving the problem at hand.

Sometimes patients say they cannot think positively, especially when chronic back pain keeps them from enjoying life and being as active as they'd like. I always tell them that just as they make choices in what to eat or what to wear, they also make the choice to think positively or negatively. They can choose to focus on the depressing, stressful aspects of life and live with the resulting negative effects on their immune systems. On the other hand, they can think positive healing thoughts that work to keep them well.

Affirmations Replace Self-Defeating Thoughts

Cognitive restructuring means replacing negative, automatic self-defeating thoughts that affect interpersonal relationships and health with more optimistic, life-affirming beliefs. It can be done, and those who have learned how to give positive statements to themselves (affirmations) throughout the day report having a better feeling about life and those around them. These affirmations should be uplifting or motivating thoughts, a short phrase or saying that has meaning and power for you.

A revealing study published in the June 2002 issue of the *Journal of Behavioral Medicine* found that pessimistic people report more pain and worse functioning than those with similar problems and a less negative outlook. While this particular study was performed on patients with knee pain, the same outcome holds true for those with back pain—or any type of chronic pain. That's because how you view life—your outlook—truly affects your health. I've seen in my patients that a negative outlook often worsens physical problems.

In this particular study, researchers measured physical pain, functioning, and outlook in 480 arthritis patients who were at least sixty-five years old. The patients all had a certain amount of disability with pain on most days. Personal outlook on life was measured by asking the participants to assess how much they agreed with optimistic statements or pessimistic statements.

The researchers reported that pessimistic participants were less able than their optimistic counterparts were to perform all of the measured daily activities such as getting in and out of a car, lifting, and walking. Researchers concluded that because pessimistic people don't think things will work out for them, they are guarded in what they do and never take risks to achieve anything. Contrary to this, optimistic people may be more likely to try new things like different exercises or positive lifestyle changes, thinking that it could really help their situation.

If you are overly pessimistic because of long-term back pain, it's important to realize that your attitude may be impacting your health. You can work on changing your negative thoughts by creating daily affirmations. Use the following steps:

1. Select an aspect of life that is causing you chronic stress, such as your back pain, family life, work responsibilities, a negative coworker or friend, financial situation, or other.
2. Decide what you'd like to have happen or how you'd rather feel in this situation such as more positive, calm, peaceful, contentment, or other.
3. Articulate this goal as a first-person, positive statement: "I am healthy and strong." Or, "I am a productive employee."
4. Repeat this affirmation many times throughout your day to help reverse negative thinking.

Here are a few examples of affirmations that can help you get through the day without allowing negativity to control your thoughts. Get in the habit of using affirmations frequently, and you'll find that your mood will improve and stressful situations will not seem overwhelming:

- I can do this.
- I like myself just as I am.
- I am calm and peaceful.
- I am physically healthy and strong.
- I love to exercise, stretch, and move around.
- I feel good about myself.

Worry Too Much? Hit the Gym

At the American Psychological Society's annual meeting in New Orleans in June 2002, researchers presented a report that chronic worriers appeared to be less likely to suffer depressive symptoms if they exercised than if they didn't exercise. Although the study was performed on students during final exam week, researchers affirmed that the findings should apply to all worriers: exercise is the treatment for worrying.

A chronic worrier is someone who worries about every situation in life—work, family, recreation activities, and more. If this describes you, block the effect worry can have on your health—and back pain—by doing something positive, that is, working out at the gym. Not only will exercise ease your emotional woes, it will help to strengthen those crucial back and abdominal muscles that can keep you pain-free.

Mind-Body Therapies Increase Well-Being

Most relaxation therapies such as progressive muscle relaxation (page 136) and biofeedback (page 141) are based on the premise that the mind and body are interrelated, and physical health and emotional well-being are closely linked. Relaxation therapy has been shown to increase the brain's morphine-like pain relievers, endorphins and enkephalins, which are associated with a happy, positive feeling. These hormones can help relay "stop-pain" messages to the body. Relaxation therapy may also improve your quality of sleep. One small study of several different relaxation procedures found a 42 percent improvement in self-reported sleep complaints after one year of relaxation therapy.

Although you cannot change life's interruptions that cause you stress, you can alter your personal reaction. Mind-body tools will give you back some control over stressful events, and many of my patients report experiencing benefits from these tools within minutes of using them. For example, deep abdominal breathing actually alters your psychological state, making a stressful moment diminish in intensity. Think about how your respiration quickens when you are fearful. Then consider how taking a deep, slow breath brings an immediate calming effect. Likewise, music therapy can lessen your heart rate in the first experience, if you mindfully block out all other "noise" and focus on the music, rhythm, and resulting inner peace.

I've found the following mind-body relaxation therapies to be useful with back pain patients. After reading Step 5, select the relaxation therapy that fits best for you and your lifestyle. This is done by trial and error, including:

1. Try the therapies explained below.
2. Record in your Pain-Free Back Diary how you feel after doing the exercise.
3. Incorporate the therapy that works best to ease your tension in your daily relaxation regimen.

The Relaxation Response
The relaxation response is a physical state of deep rest that changes the physical and emotional responses to stress. This physiological state is inborn in all of us and can at times occur when you are not aware of it.

Harvard Medical School doctor Herbert Benson first described the relaxation response more than twenty years ago. He realized that if you could induce the relaxation response at will, there was a real potential to reduce physical strain and emotional negative thoughts—and increase your ability to self-manage stress. Through his years of studies, we know that the relaxation response can be learned and certain techniques can elicit this state, such as:

Deep abdominal breathing	Repetitive prayer
Meditation	Yoga postures
Mindfulness	Visualization
Repetitive exercise	

Regular elicitation of the relaxation response can build a resiliency in dealing with stress. To induce the relaxation response, you develop an inner quiet and peacefulness, calming all negative thoughts and worries, and move your mental focus away from worries, problems, and the back pain itself. This state of relaxation offers a real potential to reduce physical strain and emotional negative thoughts—and increase your ability to self-manage pain and stress, which has a positive effect on your health and well-being. Studies show that the relaxation response slows down the sympathetic nervous system leading to

- Decreased heart rate
- Decreased blood pressure

- Decreased sweat production
- Decreased oxygen consumption
- Decreased catecholamine production (dopamine and norepineph-rine or brain chemicals associated with the stress response)
- Decreased cortisol production (stress hormone)

Learn the Relaxation Response
Set aside a period of about 20 minutes that you can devote to relaxation practice. Remove outside distractions that can disrupt your concentration: turn off the radio, the television, even the ringer on the telephone, if need be. Let family members know you want 20 minutes of quiet time and don't want to be disturbed.

1. Lie flat on a bed or floor, or recline comfortably so that your whole body is supported, relieving as much tension or tightness in your muscles as you can. You can use a pillow or cushion under your knees, if this helps to alleviate pressure on your lower back.
2. During the 20-minute period, remain as still as possible; focus your thoughts on the immediate moment, and eliminate any outside worries, which may compete for your attention.
3. As you go through these steps, in your own way try to imagine that every muscle in your body is now becoming loose, relaxed, and free of any excess tension. Picture all of the muscles in your body beginning to unwind; imagine them beginning to go loose and limp.
4. Concentrate on making your breathing even. As you exhale, picture your muscles becoming even more relaxed, as if you somehow are breathing the tension away. At the end of 20 minutes, take a few moments to study and focus on the feelings and sensations you have been able to achieve. Notice whether areas that felt tight and tense at first now feel more loose and relaxed, and whether any areas of tension or tightness remain.

4 Relaxation-Response Self-Care Techniques

1. *Deep abdominal breathing.* If you are a chest breather, taking shallow, rapid breaths can hinder relaxation. Think of a time when you felt yourself gasping for breath during an intense emotional state. Anger, fear, sadness, and even back pain can cause us to chest-breathe, making the emotional response intense. In contrast, taking slow, deep "abdominal" breaths from

the diaphragm not only oxygenates the brain, it helps to end the stress cycle and enables your heart rate and blood pressure to return to normal.

During deep abdominal breathing, you will slow down your heart rate, lower blood pressure, increase oxygen to the blood, and gain a feeling of self-control. Breathing deeply from the diaphragm also causes your body to release endorphins, while decreasing the release of stress hormones.

According to the American Institute of Stress, the quickest way to trigger the body's relaxation response any time of day is to inhale slowly. Here's how to put this method into practice:

Learn Deep Abdominal Breathing

1. Lie on your back in a quiet room with no distractions. Prop pillows under your knees to take pressure off your lower back.
2. Place your hands on your abdomen, and take in a slow, deliberate deep breath through your nostrils. If your hands are rising and your abdomen is expanding, then you are breathing correctly. If your hands do not rise, yet you see your chest rising, you are breathing incorrectly.
3. Inhale to a count of five, pause for three seconds, and then exhale to a count of five. Start with 10 repetitions of this exercise, and then increase to 25, twice daily.

Did You Know That . . .

- Stress is America's number one health problem, costing the economy more than 300 billion annually, according to the American Institute of Stress?
- Even at the lowest levels, chronic stress and anxiety result in muscle tension, which can lead to back pain, body aches, and muscle twitches?
- Levels of the stress hormone cortisol are at their highest early in the morning, making you more likely to overreact?
- Watching the late-night news can elevate your anxiety level, making it tough to fall asleep?
- People who are anxious drink and eat more?
- Anxiety increases the chance of accidents, colds, heart attacks, and back pain?

2. *Progressive muscle relaxation.* This mind-body exercise involves concentrating on different muscle groups as you contract, then relax, all of major muscle groups in the body, beginning with head, neck, arms, to chest, back, stomach, pelvis, legs, and feet. One way to use this exercise effectively for stress reduction is to do it before you get out of bed in the morning and again before you close your eyes for sleep at night. In a 2002 study at the University of Southern Mississippi, 46 volunteers who were taught progressive muscle relaxation experienced a significant dip in heart rates, perceived stress, and levels of the hormone cortisol. Cortisol changes the way the immune system functions.

To do this relaxation exercise, focus on each set of muscles, tense these muscles to the count of 10, then release to the count of 10. Along with progressive muscle relaxation, it is important to perform deep abdominal breathing, inhaling while tensing the muscles, and breathing out or exhaling while relaxing them.

3. *Visualization.* Visualization (or guided imagery) is a stress-release activity that you can do wherever you are, any time of the day or night. Imagery is a flow of thoughts you can see, hear, feel, smell, or taste or an inner representation of your experience or fantasies. This is one way your mind codes, stores, and expresses information. Imagery is also the language of emotions and the deeper self. Using visualization or imagery, you can allow your imagination to take over as you focus on your senses to create a desired state of relaxation in your mind.

Learn Visualization
Find a quiet place where you will not be disturbed. Allow 15 minutes for this exercise.

1. Lie down in a comfortable position. Prop pillows under your legs to take pressure off your back. If this is still uncomfortable, sit in a chair with good back support. Close your eyes, and take several deep breaths.
2. Imagine a peaceful place. This might be somewhere you've visited so you can have a mental picture of it. Perhaps this is the seashore at sunset or sunrise, a mountain cabin next to a babbling brook or floating on a raft in the lake on a sunny day.
3. Continue to breathe deeply and slowly, and keep this image in your mind. As you explore your mental picture of your relaxing spot,

imagine all the stress, worries, and tension leaving your body. Feel the temperature of your special place. See the colors surrounding you. What sounds do you hear? Smell the freshness of the air. Touch the gentleness of the moment. Take in all the sensory details of your relaxing place and continue to de-stress.

4. After about fifteen minutes, slowly open your eyes and acclimate yourself to the surroundings in the room. Stretch your arms and legs; gently move your head from side to side and feel the tension release. Carry the calm feeling you now have with you through the day.

4. *Meditation.* Meditation is an excellent mind-body therapy in which you focus your mind on one thought, phrase, or prayer for a certain period of time. Mindfulness meditation is a process of purposefully paying attention to what is happening in the present moment without being distracted by what has already happened or what might happen. When you do this, it leads to the relaxation response in the body, which can help to decrease heart rate, blood pressure, respiratory rate, and muscle tension. Meditation also decreases hormones such as cortisol and adrenaline, which are released during the "fight or flight" response (also called the stress response, discussed on page 122).

Meditation can guide you beyond the negative thoughts and agitations of the busy mind and allow you to become "unstuck" from your fear and other disturbing emotions. Once you've learned how to meditate effectively, you can switch into this relaxation state at will—before stressors cause you to be overwhelmed.

Learn to Meditate
Allow 15 to 20 minutes a day in your meditation sessions to see benefits.

1. Sit in a comfortable chair in a quiet room. Make sure there are no distractions. Close your eyes as you begin to meditate.
2. Focus your attention on the repetition of a word, sound, phrase or prayer; this silently or whisper. An alternative is to focus on the sensation of each breath as it moves in and out of your body.
3. Every time you notice that your attention has wandered (which will occur naturally), gently redirect it back, without judging yourself. If you continue to practice, you will learn how to meditate correctly.

8 Daily Stress Busters

1. Organize your work before you do anything else. Write down a list of priorities for the day and keep these next to your workstation.
2. Don't try to be perfect. Perfectionism will cause you more problems than not—and you will never achieve it anyway.
3. Don't feel as if you have to do everything. Share the chores. Delegate responsibilities.
4. Realize that it's okay to be "good enough." Say this aloud: "I am only one." When the pressure cooker of life begins to explode, remember that you are one person. We can do the best possible or be "good enough," but we also have to also realize our humanness and allow for this.
5. Stop multitasking. While this is a trend in American today, it will only add to your list of stressors. Do one thing at a time and mindfully focus on what you're doing. You will get more accomplished because you do it right the first time.
6. Exercise and move around more. Studies are now suggesting that exercise is even better than some pills for fighting anxiety and depression.
7. Take a leisurely bath before bedtime. A warm bath relieves muscle tension, eases aching joints, and helps your body feel relaxed before sleep.
8. Get ample sleep. Sleep deprivation is a stressor in itself since sleep restores the energy you need to better manage your back pain. Sleep also rejuvenates your joints to decrease pain and swelling. Aiming for 7 to 8 hours of sleep each night is a worthy goal as you strive to reduce excess tension that might trigger back pain.

Use Yoga

Yoga can help relieve stress and muscular tension that result in back pain. In a 2002 study, published in the journal *Work*, researchers found that regularly practicing yoga on the job helps employees to remember to use relaxation techniques to reduce stress and risks of work-related injury.

Snooze You Can Use

Pain is a foremost reason for insomnia. Some patients find back pain makes it hard to get into a comfortable position and fall asleep, while others wake up during the night and are unable to get back to sleep again. In a 1996 National Sleep Foundation survey, 65 percent of those with pain and sleep problems said that they were awakened during the night by pain. In addition, 62 percent woke up too early because of pain.

When back pain flares, getting sound sleep may cause even more stress for you. However, disrupted sleep not only affects how you feel physically, it can create a weakened emotional state. Especially as you move into your late thirties and beyond, sleep problems become a reality. Beyond age thirty-five, the efficiency of our sleep decreases as we spend less and less time in bed actually sleeping.

Many of my pain patients have experienced nonrestorative sleep, such as insomnia or light and unrefreshing sleep. New findings indicate that disordered sleep leads to lower levels of serotonin in the brain, which can result in an increase in pain sensitivity. Serotonin is a naturally occurring neurotransmitter in the body. Neurotransmitters are brain chemicals that send specific messages from one brain cell to another. What this means to those with back pain is that getting plenty of healing sleep may be an effective tool in controlling pain.

If you have difficulty sleeping because of too much stress or nagging back pain, consider these sleep suggestions:

- *Use one of the mind-body therapies discussed in this step to elicit the relaxation response when you lie down in bed.* Then, when you close your eyes for sleep, your attempt to fall asleep will not be as difficult. If you awaken during the night, use the relaxation response again to calm down and put your body back into a calm, peaceful mode.
- *Sleep only as much as you need to feel refreshed, but no more.* Some people lose sleep all week, and then try to make up for it on the weekend. This only disrupts your body's circadian rhythms. Circadian rhythms are individually synchronized internal cycles that affect our daily sleep cycles, performance and alertness, moods, and even gastrointestinal functions.
- *Wake up at the same time every day, weekday or weekend.* This strengthens your circadian cycle and will help to establish regular sleep patterns.

- *Use earplugs if you are bothered by noise while sleeping.* Some people find that "white noise"—from a machine that produces a humming sound or a radio station that has gone off the air—helps.
- *Hunger may disrupt your sleep.* Eat a snack high in serotonin-boosting carbohydrates to lull you to dreamland. Try crackers, a bagel, cereal, or frozen yogurt to relax.
- *Caffeine disturbs sound sleep.* Avoid caffeine after noon of each day.
- *Avoid alcohol.* It may seem that alcohol helps you to sleep, but it actually produces a light, fragmented sleep. Many people tell of waking up in the middle of the night after a drink or two.
- *Exercise regularly.* Avoid exercising late in the day, since it might stimulate you and make falling asleep difficult.
- *Avoid daytime napping, if you have trouble sleeping at night.* If you need to rest, sit up in a chair and listen to music or read a book. Naps can disturb sleep at nighttime.
- *Try chamomile tea, passionflower, or valerian to decrease anxiety.* These natural remedies (described on page 84) have helped some patients feel drowsy at bedtime.
- *If these therapies do not work, talk to your doctor.* Your medication could be keeping you from getting sound sleep, and sometimes changing the dosage or type of medication can enable you to feel drowsy again.

Music Therapy

Music therapy, listening to calming music for relaxation, is an excellent way to lessen stress. We know that music has a significant effect on our respiration rate, pain reduction, and anxiety levels. Music therapy can be active, such as playing the drums or piano, or passive as you listen to your favorite CD while lying down. Music is also a great way to pass the time during exercise, helping you to stay focused on the movement.

At the Tenth World Congress on Pain in 2002, renowned Australian researchers presented convincing findings on the effect of relaxation therapies and music on a patient's pain response. In the study, 65 hospitalized patients with chronic lower back pain after disk surgery were randomly divided into two groups. Both groups of patients received medical care and physical therapy, but one group also received instruction on how to use relaxation imagery while listening to soothing music.

The "relaxation" intervention group listened to music each day for 25 minutes using headphones. After three weeks, the relaxation group reported significantly improved relief from back pain, along with fewer sleep disturbances than the group who did not listen to the music.

Researchers attributed the success of relaxation therapy combined with music to a reduction in muscle tension. Both relaxation therapy and music work on the autonomic nervous system, resulting in calmness and pain reduction. Using a combination of relaxation therapies, you might be able to take less medication and still be pain-free.

Biofeedback

Centuries ago, Eastern mystics used biofeedback techniques via intense concentration to control their skin temperature, blood pressure, heart rate, and other involuntary functions. Today, biofeedback is used to teach people how to sense and control such body functions as skin temperature, heart rate, and brain waves.

Essentially any bodily process that can be measured can be potentially controlled through biofeedback. It is especially effective in relieving many pain problems as well as anxiety. The main concept of biofeedback centers on the idea that you may not be able to control what goes on around you, but you can learn to alter the way you respond to it. Biofeedback is "bio" because of biological monitoring; it is "feedback" when information from your body is returned to the source observer.

In biofeedback you are connected to a machine that informs you and your therapist when you are physically relaxing your body. With sensors placed over specific muscle sites, the therapist will read the tension in your muscles, heart rate, breathing pattern, the amount of sweat produced, or body temperature. Any one or all of these readings can let the therapist know if you are learning to relax.

The ultimate goal of biofeedback is to use this newly learned skill outside the therapist's office when you are facing the real lions and tigers of life. If learned successfully, biofeedback can help you control your heart rate, blood pressure, breathing patterns, and muscle tension when you are *not* hooked up to the machine.

The latest trend in biofeedback is to monitor your stress level throughout your workday—instead of waiting until you're completely stressed out and meditate or elicit the relaxation response. For example, at some major corporations, employees can literally plug in to their desktop computer to take a read of their stress levels.

Employees use a finger clip to hook themselves up to a biofeedback monitor on their PC, which uses a software program called Freeze-Framer. The program measures heart rhythms and gives a reading on how the body is handling stress at that moment.

It does take time to learn biofeedback and even longer to learn to use it outside the therapist's office. Some people get results in just three or four sessions. A full treatment varies from twelve to twenty treatments.

Some common types of biofeedback include:

- *Electromyographic (EMG) biofeedback.* Provides feedback on muscle tension and works well for patients with anxiety disorders or chronic pain.
- *Electrodermal (EDR) biofeedback.* Measures subtle changes in amounts of perspiration.
- *Thermal biofeedback.* The temperature of the skin is measured and results are used in teaching hand warming. This has been found to help relieve migraine headaches and can benefit those with Raynaud's disease.
- *Finger pulse biofeedback.* The finger pulse records heart rate and force and is useful for anxiety or cardiovascular symptoms.
- *Respiration biofeedback.* This type of biofeedback shows the rate, volume, rhythm, and location of each breath.

Hypnosis

Hypnosis is yet another successful mind-body therapy to modulate back pain. This intense state of concentration is used to control pain, stress, and sleep problems or to alter negative behaviors. Even experts are unsure as to how hypnosis works to resolve pain, but it is thought that hypnosis changes your expectations about how intense the pain will be, which alters the pain you actually feel. It may also be that when you focus your attention on a competing image, this helps to block your perception of back pain. The ultimate goal of hypnosis is to be able to manage your own pain.

With hypnosis, you concentrate deeply on a single thought. The therapist may also use role-playing, imagination, motivation, and the power of suggestion in this therapy to enhance the session. Hypnosis requires you to truly desire to change a type of behavior. In fact, success might be greater in those who are desperate to change behaviors.

It is thought that only about 15 percent of the population may be "highly hypnotizable," and 25 percent are thought to be not hypnotizable at all. According to the American Association of Professional Hypnotherapists, there is a 75 to 90 percent chance of changing behavior with hypnotherapy. If you consider hypnosis, it's important to note that the success of your outcome depends greatly on the practitioner's experience and expertise, as well as your willingness to change.

Integrating Mind-Body Therapies

Your particular patterns of muscle tension are learned responses—not something that is part of your genetic makeup. In other words, each time life's stressors hit, you have learned to respond by tightening your muscles, clenching your jaw, or furrowing your brow. For those with chronic back pain, the excess tension felt when back pain flares may be something you can control—and greatly reduce. For example, my patient Beverly met with a biofeedback therapist for six weeks and was amazed to find how she held her tension in her shoulders, neck, and back, particularly during times of stress.

"I'm such a perfectionist in every way, and if things were the least bit out of order or not according to my plan, I would respond by tightening the muscles in my body," Beverly said. "The therapist helped me to identify this learned tension response. Once I was confronted with it, I started learning how to change it. For instance, I've learned to talk more about my feelings instead of stuffing the emotions inside and holding tension, which always resulted in chronic back pain. I now exercise more, since it's hard to feel tense if I'm walking on my treadmill or planting flowers in my garden. I also do yoga postures each morning when I awaken, before my busy day begins, and take several breaks throughout the day to practice the relaxation exercises. All of these practices have helped me to soothe myself and relax, and my back pain has improved dramatically."

Beverly is an excellent example of how you can release tension and anxiety as you change your stress response and look at life's problems more positively. As you become more aware of your body and how you respond to stress, use this four-point technique to become aware of what's increasing your stress and choose a positive response:

1. *Stop* when stressors begin to make you feel anxious and overwhelmed.
2. *Breathe* from your diaphragm to the count of 10.

3. *Relax* your muscles throughout your body as you change your response.
4. *Respond* in an upbeat manner as you focus on positive affirmations instead of ruminating on life's interruptions.

As you probably know by now, stress will never go away. There will always be one more interruption, predicament, or crisis that will vie for your emotional reaction. However, how you respond to life's stressors can make all the difference in your back pain and overall health. The mind-body suggestions in this step will let you become a more positive, productive person in all facets of life and keep your back healthy for life.

Pain-Free Back Mind-Body Rx

- Realizing that stress and tension contribute to back pain, assess your daily stressors. Write these down in your Pain-Free Back Diary.
- Review the stress symptoms, outlined on page 122. If you have any of these symptoms, talk to your doctor about ways to resolve them before they injure your physical or emotional health.
- Write affirmations about yourself, and use these daily to overcome negative or critical thinking patterns.
- Review the various mind-body therapies given in this step and attempt to try each one several times. Write down in your diary how you feel after doing a particular therapy.
- Learn to organize your life, setting priorities on what's important and what's not. Practice saying no if you are asked to overextend yourself.
- Review the "Snooze You Can Use" on page 139, and work on your sleep hygiene.

Healing Touch Therapies

Forty-eight-year-old Nancy had been fighting back pain for years. Not only did she have a herniated disk but fibromyalgia and osteoarthritis had created such a painful back condition that she was considering stopping her job as a paralegal at large law firm.

After evaluating Nancy's combination of back problems, I recommended that she immediately start the regular exercise, moist heat, and other therapies in my *Pain-Free Back Program*. Using this combination of complementary treatments, Nancy would get fast pain relief, so she could be more active and continue working full-time. I then suggested that she have a regular massage as adjunct therapy, especially since her day job entailed long hours of sitting at a computer workstation. Because Nancy suffers the deep muscle pain of fibromyalgia, I specifically recommended neuromuscular therapy (see page 150). (At this time, the American Academy of Pain Management recognizes this form of massage therapy as an effective treatment for back pain caused by soft tissue injury, such as a muscle strain.)

Within a month of starting the *Pain-Free Back Program* and having regular neuromuscular therapy sessions, Nancy was sold on the complementary approach to treatment. "I feel great. I look forward to Friday evening when I have the one-hour massage. Then I am able to be even more active over the weekend because my pain and stiffness are greatly reduced," she said. "Along with the massage, my therapist helps me with my Pain-Free Back stretches and range-of-motion exercises. She also uses moist heat on my lower back to ease pain and inflammation when I'm tense."

Often tagged as "drug-free doctoring," massage is an excellent complementary therapy because it views the mind and body as a totally integrated system. This means they influence each other and depend on your total participation in self-care to stay well. Massage influences all body systems, from circulation and the nervous system to digestion, emotions, and more. Using complementary therapies such as massage to end back pain has its advantages, since you can often take fewer medications and avoid the potential side effects of some drugs.

If you want to try healing touch therapies to ease your back pain, I recommend several in this step. Depending on the nature of your problem, one of these hands-on healing modalities can surely boost the positive results you're now getting from Steps 1 to 5 of the *Pain-Free Back Program*. While I would not advise you to use any single manual therapy as the only treatment for back pain, I do know that when touch therapies are combined with a multifaceted program of exercise, moist heat, diet and lifestyle changes, and medication, you can almost guarantee optimum relief of pain and stiffness. Especially with the soaring costs of health care, complementary touch treatments, which range from massage to Pilates to acupuncture, are relatively affordable, easily accessible, and allow you to participate actively in key decisions about your health.

Caution

If you have severe lower back pain, redness, or inflammation, it is advisable to check with your personal physician before beginning massage therapy.

Pain-Free Back Manual Touch Therapies

Alexander Technique	Physical therapy
Backrub	Pilates
Chiropractic	Polarity therapy
Deep tissue massage	Reiki
Feldenkrais	Rolfing Structural Integration
Hellerwork	Shiatsu
Movement integration	Structural alignment
Neuromuscular massage	Swedish massage
Osteopathy	Trager Method

Bodywork

Bodywork (also called manual healing therapy) is the umbrella term that refers to a variety of body manipulation therapies used for relaxation and pain relief. Massage and chiropractic are well-known forms of bodywork, along with Pilates, Rolfing, Alexander Technique, and Trager Method. Bodywork is often used as a complementary therapy to relieve muscle tension and spasms, promote relaxation, and reduce pain from ailments such as fibromyalgia and arthritis.

Understanding Massage Therapy

The basic philosophy of massage therapy is to help the body to heal itself, and in doing so, increase health and well-being. The fundamental medium of massage therapy is human touch with various manual techniques—gliding, rubbing, kneading, tapping, manipulating, holding, friction pressure, taping, and vibrating—using primarily the hands. Massage therapists may also use their knuckles, forearms, elbows, or even their feet to help normalize the body. These techniques affect the musculoskeletal, circulatory-lymphatic, nervous, and other bodily systems.

How it works. As the therapist manipulates the body's soft tissue structures it improves function of the circulatory, muscular, skeletal and nervous systems and stimulates the body's lymph system to carry wastes and impurities away from tissues. Many of my patients find that this therapy, when combined with regular exercise, moist heat and other strategies in the *Pain-Free Back Program*, helps to alleviate back pain. In fact, in a study on back pain conducted at the Touch Research Institute at the University of Miami, researchers concluded that massage lessened lower back pain, depression and anxiety, and improved sleep. The massage therapy group in the study showed improved range of motion and their serotonin and dopamine levels were higher. Dopamine is often referred to as the brain's "pleasure chemical" because of its role in transmitting signals related to pleasurable experiences. Serotonin is a brain neurotransmitter that is involved in generating feelings of well-being and satisfaction.

Some researchers believe the hormone oxytocin gets a boost after a massage. Oxytocin is best known for its role in inducing labor and is tagged the "quintessential maternal hormone." When it is released into the brain, it is known to promote calming and positive social behaviors. In humans, oxytocin stimulates milk ejection during lactation, uterine contraction during birth, and is released during sexual orgasm in both men and women. These new studies show that increased levels of oxytocin can reduce cortisol levels, ease anxiety, and positively affect relationships.

In a revealing study published in the journal *Psychiatry*, researchers measured oxytocin levels in twenty-five women. In the study, researchers found that blood levels of the hormone oxytocin rose significantly following neck and shoulder massages. Because chronic elevation of the stress hormone cortisol is a predictor for early-onset hypertension and other chronic diseases, reducing cortisol may help you live longer, feel healthier, and even improve your pain response.

Back pain benefits. Massage therapy gives relief from lower back pain and may increase joint mobility, decrease muscle stiffness and spasms, and improve circulation, which aids in recovery of muscle soreness from physical activity or injury. Massage also increases relaxation, which can help to calm anxiety and improve sleep problems. Some new studies have shown that massage alters the sleep pattern, which reduces levels of the chemical messenger for pain, substance P.

With massage, the brain boosts the production of enkephalins and their related chemicals endorphins, which are part of the brain's painkiller and stress-response system. These chemicals regulate and suppress painful or stress-related signals in the brain.

Choosing a therapist. The Commission on Massage Training Accreditation (COMTA) is one of the main regulatory institutions for the massage therapy industry. A majority of the states regulate massage therapists and require 500 hours of instruction before being offered a license. A registered massage therapist must hold the appropriate diploma, certificate, or equivalent from an accredited vocational massage therapy school.

Associated Bodywork and Massage Professionals (ABMP) provides professional support and legislative advocacy for massage therapists and bodyworkers. Membership is at two levels: practitioner level requires 100 hours of training. Professional level requires 500 hours. ABMP also publishes *Massage and Bodywork Quarterly*.

Contraindications to Massage Therapy

Inflammation of the veins	Some skin conditions
Infectious diseases	Certain cardiac problems
Certain types of cancer	

How to Give a Back Rub

If you have low back pain that responds to touch therapies, talk a family member or friend into giving you a soothing back rub to increase circulation and relaxation. Here are some tips:

1. Have the person lie face down on a comfortable mat. Apply a light massage oil such as sesame, lavender, patchouli, or lemon to the back. Starting at the person's lower back or waist, begin to apply gentle, gliding strokes in the direction of blood flow to the heart. As you apply pressure to the back, push toward the heart and put less pressure on the return stroke.
2. Using your fingers, massage the muscle by making tiny circles that go deeper into the skin than the initial gliding strokes.
3. Using a brisk stroke across the skin, rub the area to be massaged to warm it up.
4. Massage deeper into the muscle, continuing with the gliding strokes. Use the palm of the hand or fingertips.
5. Finish with gliding strokes that are soothing and gentle. Pat the back dry with a soft towel. Or, to ease pain and stiffness, apply a moist heating pad to the person's back for 15 minutes.

Popular Massage Therapies

Lori's story is one you might relate to: a dancer as a young adult, three young children before age thirty, a sedentary career as a stenographer, a weight gain of thirty-five pounds since college, and now inactive because of low back pain. Lori said her back hurt "all day, every day," until she started the *Pain-Free Back Program*. She had been extremely fit as a dancer but now she had a hard time picking up her two-year-old because she was so out of shape. When she first started the exercises discussed in Step 1, Lori admitted she could only do a few stretches before feeling fatigued and sore.

I suggested that Lori consider adding an hour-long massage treatment to her program. As a busy mother, she was excited about massage for stress reduction, as well as pain relief. Within three weeks of having this therapy, Lori was able to exercise more and with much less pain. When I saw her three months later, she said massage helped her move from being "overfat and underfit" to getting back in shape, losing weight, and ending her nagging backache. Lori now sleeps soundly at night because she's not in pain and has increased energy the next day to enjoy her family, career, and exercise program.

Several types of massage are commonly performed in the United States, including the four that follow.

Swedish massage. Of all massage techniques, Swedish massage is the most popular. This style of hands-on touch uses effleurage, a stroking style that is very rhythmic and synchronized. Swedish massage also involves long strokes, kneading and friction on the surface layer of muscles, and movement of the joints. It is combined with active and passive movements of the joints, and oil is usually used, which facilitates the stroking and kneading of the body, thereby stimulating metabolism and circulation. The therapist applies pressure and rubs the muscles in the same direction as the flow of blood returning to the heart. Swedish massage is said to help flush the tissue of lactic and uric acids and other metabolic wastes, as well as to improve circulation without increasing the load on the heart.

Neuromuscular massage. A common form of massage for back pain is Neuromuscular Therapy (NT), also called trigger-point therapy. This type of massage focuses on spots where muscle fibers, damaged by exertion or tension, have adhered to each other or to surrounding tissue or bone, causing the fibers to no longer extend and contract properly. By combining basic principles of Oriental pressure therapies along with a specific hands-on deep tissue therapy, the therapist can help reduce chronic muscle or myofascial (soft tissue) pain and muscle spasms.

Neuromuscular massage is applied specifically to individual muscles and is used to increase blood flow, release trigger points (intense knots of muscle tension that refer pain to other parts of the body), and release pressure on nerves caused by soft tissues. Shiatsu and acupressure are common forms of trigger-point therapy or neuromuscular massage.

Deep tissue massage. This type of massage is applied with greater pressure and at deeper layers of the muscle than Swedish massage and is used to release chronic patterns of muscular tension using slow strokes, direct pressure, or friction. Often the movements are directed across the grain of the muscles (cross-fiber) using the fingers, thumbs, or elbows. Hellerwork (see page 151) is an example of deep tissue massage.

Movement Integration. This technique involves deep massage that works to realign the body by changing the length and tone of certain tissues. Based on the premise that most humans are significantly out of alignment with gravity, movement integration promotes natural healing by realigning the body's underlying structure. The practitioner uses fingers, knuckles, and elbows to "sculpt" the client's body into correct alignment. This deep pressure helps to stretch the muscles and *fascia,* thick elastic connective tissue that envelops and supports muscles, tendons and bones, making them more flexible.

How Massage Affects the Body

A 30-minute massage can influence:

- The nervous system
- The musculoskeletal system
- The cardiovascular system
- The respiratory system
- The digestive system
- The lymphatic system

Specific Types of Bodywork

Alexander Technique. More than a century old, the Alexander Technique can help reeducate the mind and body to make you aware of your total movement patterns—from sitting to standing to lifting to lying still. The technique helps to relieve back pain and prevent recurrences by correcting poor posture and teaching proper movement techniques. It can release painful muscle tension, improve posture, and reduce stress and fatigue through reeducation of the kinesthetic sense. Because you are an active participant, you will learn to reeducate yourself to effectively change bad habits.

Feldenkrais. Using a series of subtle movements to help you increase range of motion, the Feldenkrais practitioner focuses on improving your flexibility, coordination, and movement with hands-on communication. Feldenkrais is well-known for its ability to improve posture and flexibility and alleviate muscular tension and pain through a unique method of moving, sitting, standing that enables your body to work with gravity instead of against it. A series of lessons will teach you how to improve your posture and become flexible and spontaneous. Subconscious holding patterns are brought to your awareness, then you are shown how to release these to reclaim a healthy mind-body connection.

Hellerwork. The basic principle of Hellerwork is to realign the body through manipulation. This touch therapy is effective for acute back pain or tension relief and can also help to improve posture. With Hellerwork, a trained practitioner combines hands-on massage, movement, and conversation to help you release accumulated stress and rigidity. Rather than treating the "symptom," such as muscle tension or pain, Hellerwork practitioners focus on rebalancing the entire body, returning it to a more aligned, relaxed, and youthful state.

Polarity Therapy. This form of bodywork is based on the theory that energy fields exist everywhere in nature, including in the human body. Stress, tension, chronic pain, and environmental stimuli are among many factors that can restrict this energy flow, causing disease. The polarity therapist will use gentle body manipulation and holding of pressure points to help restore natural energy flow. The therapist will also educate you in exercise, nutrition, and maintaining a positive attitude to keep energy fields balanced.

Reiki. Based on the same energetic principles as tai chi and acupuncture, Reiki is neither invasive nor physical. Practitioners believe that the vital energy of the universe is channeled through their hands to help energize you and promote inner healing. Proponents claim that Reiki has a calming effect and can restore balance to the body. During a Reiki session, you will stay clothed and lie on your back on a massage table. The Reiki healer will gently rest her hands on various parts of the body in patterns, which include the head, abdomen, legs, back, and feet. You may feel a sensation of warmth during this treatment, which usually takes about an hour.

Rolfing. Rolfing is an example of structural integration. According to this philosophy of manual therapy, poor posture influences our physical and emotional well-being. This causes a disorganized body that demands increased energy in order to keep an upright position. Over time, the body becomes imbalanced and serious posture problems result in pain and distress.

The Rolfer aims to realign the body by movement integration with deep manipulation of connective tissue or fascia, which is aimed at relieving physical misalignment and letting the body correct itself. Once the muscles and connective tissues are balanced, the body functions optimally and the immune system is more effective.

Rolfing can sometimes be painful because the practitioner uses firm pressure with the fingers and elbows to specific parts of the body. While the Rolfing process extends over a course of ten sessions, if you have a low pain threshold, try one session before making a commitment. Also, make sure the Rolfer is certified and trained by the Rolf Institute.

Shiatsu. A Japanese form of acupressure or acupuncture without needles, Shiatsu is different from most Western types of massage. The practitioner does not use oils or strokes that you normally associate with massage. Instead, a shiatsu practitioner uses his hands, elbows, knees, and even feet to press various points along twelve energy pathways known as meridians in order to balance energy (*Chi*, or *Qi*), which is the body's life force and critical for maintaining good health.

The meridians start at your fingertips, connect to the brain, and then connect to the organ associated with the specific meridian. The twelve major meridians correspond to specific human organs: kidneys, liver, spleen, heart, lungs, pericardium, bladder, gallbladder, stomach, small and large intestines, and the triple burner (body temperature regulator).

The shiatsu practitioner applies gentle to deep pressure to specific points on the meridians, called *tsubos*. The pressure is held for several seconds and is repeated several times before the practitioner moves to another tsubo. The pressure may help to stimulate the body's endorphins to produce a tranquilizing effect, or it may help by loosening up muscles and improving blood circulation. With shiatsu, the practitioner may also use pulling and pushing strokes, tapping, rubbing, stroking, and squeezing to influence the body's tissues.

It is thought that shiatsu is based on the laws of physics or the study of motion and reaction produced by external forces. In physics, there is a law which states that when there is a force exerted on one object there is an equal and opposite force or reaction on a first object by the second. In shiatsu, when the practitioner applies stimulation to a point on the body, whether by pressing, rubbing, or kneading, the body accordingly produces some internal changes. Thus, a practitioner of these techniques applies dynamic stimulation to the patient, administering pressure rhythmically in changing degrees, so that the patient feels the multiple results of varying applications of this stimulation and pressure.

Acupressure. A form of Chinese healing, acupressure uses touch to unblock *qi* and allow the meridians or pathways to flow smoothly. Discovered before acupuncture, acupressure depends on the same bodily points but no needles are used. For example, a point on your hand might help headaches. A point on the ankle can boost liver function. An acupressure point on the wrist can stop nausea.

With this manual therapy, a practitioner uses the fingers to press key points on the surface of the skin to stimulate the body's natural self-curative abilities. Pressure is applied gently initially, but then increases to the point where a strong sensation is felt. The direction of the manual

Acupressure, Endorphins, and Pain

Researchers believe that both acupressure and acupuncture cause the body to release endorphins and monoamines, chemicals that block pain signals in the spinal cord and the brain. The endorphin system consists of chemicals that regulate the activity of a group of nerve cells in the brain that relax muscles, dull pain, and reduce panic and anxiety. These ancient touch therapies may also trigger the release of more hormones, including serotonin, a brain chemical that makes you feel calm and serene, as well as the anti-inflammatory chemical known as cortisol. With acupressure, not only are you benefiting from touching the trigger points, but you also benefit from increased circulation and decreased tension.

stimulation should follow the natural flow of *qi* in the meridians. The energy point is simulated using the same finger, which helps to unblock the channels, according to proponents of acupressure.

Many have experienced that using acupressure regularly helps to trigger the relaxation response (see page 134), a physiological state characterized by a feeling of warmth and quiet mental alertness.

Trager Method. The Trager Method includes table work (a practitioner gently rocks and lengthens your body to release tension) followed by a movement lesson for continued self-care. The practitioner will use gentle to vigorous rocking movements to loosen joint restrictions and promote relaxation. Using pressure and stretching, the practitioner will help you give up muscular and mental tension and sink into a feeling of deep relaxation.

With Trager, expect to do homework, particularly a series of movements called Mentastics®, which involve shaking the joints and promotes progressively greater relaxation and freedom of movement. One of the most important aspects of Trager is that you'll learn how to recall the feeling of calmness and deep relaxation, and how it feels to move freely and easily.

Understanding Pilates

Donna, a forty-one-year-old mother and research librarian, told me that she was "tired of hurting all over" from the deep muscle pain of fibromyalgia. Faced with taking a leave from her job at a university library because of lower back and hip pain, Donna turned to Pilates (puh-LAH-teez) as a last resort to relearn how to improve her posture and use her muscles correctly.

"At first I thought Pilates was going to be something like low-impact aerobics and worsen my pain, instead of helping me heal. I admit that I was almost afraid to attend the first session. Yet, after the instructor explained the purpose of Pilates, I realized that it was a gentle body-conditioning process of learning breathing patterns and how to move each muscle properly.

"Using gentle touch, the instructor guides me through specific and sometimes intense strengthening exercises to work my torso—from the neck to lower back, including the abdominals—helping to stabilize and lengthen my spine. I do all the exercises under supervision, and it has changed my life. My muscles are stronger, and my posture and coordination are much better. I have less pain and feel more alive."

While strength training tends to shorten muscles, Pilates lengthens them. This system of strengthening and stretching exercises has come into its own in popularity, with more than five hundred studios across the nation. Devised by Joseph Pilates, a German gymnast and boxer, in the early part of the twentieth century, it was based on the concept of strengthening the body's "powerhouse," the corset of muscles around the pelvis and lower abdomen. Pilates believed that when these muscles are under strain, other joints and muscles will be stressed as well.

Today, the Pilates system works the deeper muscles to achieve efficient and graceful movement, improve alignment and breathing, and increase body awareness. You can do Pilates on a mat, or with special pieces of equipment called the Reformer, Cadillac, Wunda Chair, Pedipull, and Barrel. Proponents of Pilates claim it helps you become more aware of your posture and how you move, sit and stand, and patients like Donna are firm believers in its merit for helping to end back pain.

Many patients with chronic back pain have experienced complete recovery after learning this exercise system. Instead of working major muscle groups in isolation, Pilates works the whole body in synergy. You must think about the exercises, and it takes all your concentration. Pilates depends on personal instruction and specific machines for the exercises. Contact a studio in your area for more information.

Spinal Adjustments and Manipulation Therapies

About a year ago, twenty-nine-year-old Daniel took a hard fall while snowboarding in Colorado. Although he had no broken bones, he did damage muscles in his back, causing severe pain and stiffness. Over the course of the year, the pain subsided as Daniel used the *Pain-Free Back Program*. Yet, still feeling he needed an added boost to be completely pain-free, this young athlete turned to chiropractic and found that spinal adjustments, combined with his other therapies, helped reduce his pain and stiffness.

Chiropractic

Instead of treating the symptoms, such as lower back pain, doctors of chiropractic focus on adjusting the spine with a specific directional thrust that sets a vertebra that might have been affected by stress, trauma, or other causes into its normal position. The doctor will administer an adjustment or a specific force in a precise direction applied to a joint that is fixated, locked up, or not moving properly. Although chiropractors are not medical doctors, they are educated at accredited chiropractic colleges as health care providers with an emphasis on musculoskeletal treatment through manual and physical procedures, such as manipulation, massage, exercise, and nutrition.

How it works. According to doctors of chiropractic, your nervous system controls all functions in your body. Messages must travel from your brain down your spinal cord, then out to the nerves at particular parts of the body, and then back to the spinal cord and up to the brain. The theory is that abnormal positions of the spinal bones may interfere with these messages and are often the underlying cause of many health problems. The chiropractic doctor may also recommend a program of rehabilitation to stabilize and reduce joint involvement, rehabilitate muscle ligament tissue, and balance nerve impulses.

Back pain benefits. Chiropractic is a drug-free touch therapy that focuses on restoring and maintaining health through gentle, careful adjustments of the body joints and spine to restore normal nerve function. Chiropractic is becoming increasingly popular for treatment of acute back pain. Results of a study on more than 800 patients published in the May 2000 issue of the *Journal of the Geriatric Society* stated that more than half of people over age fifty-five seek chiropractic care for mild to moderate complaints. Musculoskeletal pain, such as lower back pain, accounts for nine out of ten chiropractic visits. Numerous other clinical studies, including randomized controlled trials, confirm the suitability of chiropractic care for lower back pain.

Osteopathy

Osteopathy is a holistic healing philosophy that emphasizes promotion of health and prevention of disease. Osteopathic physicians are trained to use a finely honed "sense of touch" to feel dysfunction in the patient's tissues. They use Osteopathic Manipulative Treatment (OMT) to relieve muscle pain and boost recovery from illness by promoting blood flow through tissues.

Developed in the late 1800s by Dr. Andrew Taylor Still, osteopathy was based on the principle of treating the body by improving its natural functions rather than using medication. Today, osteopathy is a full system of health care and medical philosophy that continues to emphasize the relationship between the body's nerves, muscles, bones, and organs, and overall health.

How it works. Doctors of osteopathy (DO) are fully licensed and trained medical doctors who have additional training in osteopathic manipulation. Diagnosing the connection is often done by moving the hands along the patient's body, feeling the body's living anatomy (that is, flow of fluids, motion and texture of tissues, and structural makeup) and looking for areas that may feel swollen or tense from chronic pain. Osteopathic physicians believe that a patient's illnesses or physical traumas are written into the body's structure.

Back pain benefits. Using a highly developed sense of touch, the osteopathic physician may be able to detect physical problems that fail to appear on X ray or other imaging tools. In a study published in the November 1999 issue of the *New England Journal of Medicine*, osteopathic manipulation was performed on 178 patients with back pain for at least three weeks but less than six months. Patients who received osteopathic manipulation had similar clinical results as those receiving conventional medical treatment in the study, with the latter group using significantly more medication and more physical therapy.

Focus on the Spine

Although there are specific differences between chiropractic and osteopathy, both of these healing disciplines are based on the idea that dislocations or malalignments of bone, specifically the spine, are a major source of pain and disease. Spinal manipulation is defined as manual loading of the spine using short or long leverage methods. This type of manual therapy is safe and sometimes effective for those who with symptoms of acute back pain. With spinal manipulation, the practitioner moves the joint beyond its normal end range of motion. You may even hear a cracking or popping sound, which often occurs with movement.

For the short term, the benefits of manual therapy may be good. In fact, chiropractic adjustments are very popular in the United States, with as many as 40 million Americans receiving regular treatment. Yet the long-term effect of manual therapy is minimal, as shown by numerous studies. For instance, a study published in the October 1998 *New England Journal of Medicine* reviewed the course of 321 adults with low back pain that persisted for more than seven days. These patients were treated with either chiropractic manipulation or a special method of physical therapy, or they were given an educational booklet on resolving back pain. At a two-year follow-up consultation, researchers found that though physical therapy and chiropractic manipulation had similar effects and costs, those patients had only slightly better outcomes than patients who received the minimal intervention of an educational booklet.

The 7 Basic Beliefs of Osteopathy

1. Health is a holistic product of mind, body, and environment.
2. The body's structure and function are linked.
3. If a body part isn't working right, it will eventually become diseased.
4. Blood circulation is essential to healing.
5. The body constantly readjusts itself to balance weak areas with strong ones.
6. The body has an innate ability to heal itself.
7. Prevention is central to health care.

Acupuncture

Acupuncture is one of the oldest, most commonly used medical procedures in the world. It is offered in many chronic pain clinics and is covered by some insurance companies. The World Health Organization (WHO) recommends acupuncture for treatment of chronic pain, and a National Institutes of Health panel concluded that acupuncture was an acceptable modality for treating musculoskeletal pain and fibromyalgia (deep muscle pain), along with other ailments.

Originating in China more than two thousand years ago, this Traditional Chinese Medicine therapy is based upon the theory of a vital energy (*Chi* or *Qi*) that circulates through the body in channels called meridians. Disease occurs when the flow of vital energy is obstructed.

With acupuncture, a practitioner inserts one or more tiny, dry needles into the skin at specific points. These points may be stimulated by pressure (acupressure), laser, ultrasound, heat (moxibustion)—counter irritation produced by igniting a cone or cylinder of moxa placed on the skin, or electricity (electroacupuncture).

How it works. To receive the treatment, you lie down on a table or sit in a chair, so the practitioner has access to the skin at specific points. The practitioner will then place the stainless steel needles into your skin at specific sites that are thought to correspond to certain organs and anatomic areas deep within the body. When the tiny needle is inserted into a specific point on the body, it stimulates nerves in the underlying muscles. According to scientists, this stimulation sends impulses up the spinal cord to the limbic system, a primitive part of the brain. The impulses also go to the midbrain and the pituitary gland. In some cases, the needles are left in place for a period of time. Usually, however, the needles are gently moved using a rotating or pumping action.

Back pain benefits. Studies have shown that acupuncture may alter brain chemistry by changing the release of neurotransmitters, the biochemical substances that stimulate or inhibit nerve impulses in the brain that relay information about external stimuli and sensations, such as pain, in a good way. Acupuncture has also been documented to affect the parts of the central nervous system related to sensation and involuntary body functions, such as immune reactions and processes whereby your blood pressure, blood flow, and body temperature are regulated. Because acupuncture is a way to stimulate nerves and muscles, some experts believe that it releases various neurotransmitters, including opioid peptides and serotonin.

If you choose to try acupuncture, make sure your practitioner is qualified and uses disposable needles. The American Academy of Medical Acupuncture (AAMA) is the sole physician-only professional acupuncture society in North America. Members must have an active license to practice medicine in the United States or Canada as a Medical Doctor or Doctor of Osteopathy. These health care professionals receive 220 hours in formal training in medical acupuncture, along with two years experience practicing medical acupuncture before they are fully eligible for membership in the AAMA. Credentials for acupuncturists have various titles, including L.Ac., Lic.Ac., C.A., Dipl.Ac., M.Ac., or AAMA.

Fast Facts

The National Institutes of Health (NIH) Consensus Conference on Acupuncture concluded that acupuncture was effective in treating certain types of pain. Approximately 14,000 practicing acupuncturists are licensed in more than forty states. This number is expected to reach 21,000 by the year 2005. Treatment consists of 6 to 12 sessions scheduled over several months, each lasting approximately 30 minutes or less.

Physical and Occupational Therapy

Physical therapy, also known as physiotherapy, and occupational therapy are integral components of back pain treatment. With physical therapy, a trained professional uses manual touch and exercises, along with heat, ice, ultrasound, and other methods to ease back pain and promote healing. For example, moist heat is frequently used to help decrease pain in a swollen or painful muscle or joint as the therapist prepares you for exercises. When used along with deep muscle massage, the benefit may include greater range of motion or increased mobility. Cold therapies, such as ice packs, can reduce muscle spasms that come from joint problems or irritated nerves. Cold is one of the treatments for pain caused by inflamed tissues and other swelling.

A physical therapist will evaluate your musculoskeletal status and review your strength, range of motion, and posture. Using a combination of exercises, posture training, and educational counseling, the therapist will help you reduce extra stress on your back during daily activities such as walking, sitting, standing, lifting, and lying down. If you work at a computer workstation all day and have chronic back pain, the physical therapist can show you proper ways to sit to maintain erect posture and keep your body from becoming imbalanced. Or if you have osteoarthritis of the spine, the physical therapist can show you how to avoid stressing the back while lifting or standing for long periods of time. Learning to live with the chronic back pain problem is important to avoid painful flares.

An occupational therapist will use interviews, observation and functional assessment to evaluate you and then plan an effective treatment plan that allows you to do daily activities and fulfill career responsibilities without further injury or pain. For instance, an occupational therapist can help you set up an ergonomically correct computer workstation. He or she can show you how to perform daily activities, including dressing, bathing, and meal preparation, without added load on the joints and muscles and without fear of injury of falling. (See more on occupational therapy and assistive devices on page 105).

Ultrasound

Ultrasound uses sound waves to help soothe painful muscles and tendons. It can be used to treat acute injuries to soft tissues or to treat soft tissue pain that has become chronic. It is safe when applied by an experienced person, and if you find relief treatment can be continued. Your physical therapist can decide if ultrasound may be helpful for your situation.

TENS and PENS

In some cases of back pain, transcutaneous electrical nerve stimulation (TENS) may be used. This older form of treatment is less commonly used today, but if you find relief from it, can be used safely.

With TENS, your physical therapist will connect you to a "TENS unit," through which you'll receive continuous pulses of electrical stimulation via four electrode pads placed on the back and connected to a small, portable battery-operated device. The pulses might feel like a mild tingling, tapping, or massaging sensation and are thought to interrupt pain impulses from the periphery to the central nervous system. It is also thought that TENS works by increasing the production of endorphins, the body's natural opioids, and improves blood supply to the painful site on the body.

Percutaneous Electrical Nerve Stimulation (PENS) is a technique that uses acupuncture-like needle probes positioned in the soft tissues and/or muscles to stimulate peripheral sensory nerves at appropriate levels. Some believe that PENS may be more effective than TENS or exercise therapy in patients with persistent back pain.

Touch Therapies Really Work

Just as other back pain treatments in Steps 1 to 5 have been put to the test in a host of clinical trials, so have many manual therapies. The results have been extremely positive:

• A study in the March 2001 *Journal of Holistic Nursing* reported on shiatsu massage as an intervention therapy for 66 adults with lower back pain. Each person's anxiety and pain levels were measured before and after four shiatsu treatments. Each subject was then called two days following each shiatsu treatment and asked to evaluate their pain level. Researchers concluded that shiatsu significantly decreased both lower back pain and anxiety over time.

• A study published in the May 1996 *Journal of Clinical and Experimental Rheumatology* revealed significant improvement in the pain rating, pain frequency, and analgesic drug consumption in adults with back pain who used a multidisciplinary approach to treatment, including Alexander Technique, chiropractic, and acupuncture. Researchers reported that patients continued to have good relief from back pain six months after the study ended.

• A study published in January 2002 in the journal *Medical Clinics of North America* concluded that massage therapy and manual techniques have usefulness, specifically as adjunct therapy to a comprehensive treatment program. Researchers found that manual techniques are especially useful for painful conditions as a means to break the pain cycle and increase tolerance of exercise and other educational approaches.

• Researchers at Ludwig-Maximilians University in Germany studied the affect of acupuncture on patients suffering with chronic neck pain, including those who had myofascial pain syndrome lasting more than five years. (Myofascial pain syndrome is muscle pain in specific areas that may be caused by physical or emotional tension). In findings published in June 2001 in the *British Medical Journal*, in just one week after receiving an acupuncture treatment, more than half of those treated with acupuncture reported a more than 50 percent improvement in pain.

• In a study at Touch Research Institute in Miami, published in the *International Journal of Neuroscience*, researchers randomly assigned twenty-four adults with lower back pain to either massage therapy or a progressive muscle relaxation group. The twice-weekly sessions lasted for five weeks. On the first and last day of the study, volunteers completed questionnaires, provided a urine sample, and were assessed for range of motion. Researchers concluded that massage therapy was the most effective in reducing pain, stress hormones, such as cortisol, and symptoms associated with chronic low back pain. Along with pain relief, participants who received massage therapy reported less depression and anxiety and that their sleep had improved. They also showed improved movement, and their serotonin and dopamine levels were higher as measured by laboratory testing.

Make an Appointment Today

Will manual touch work for your back pain? Can a regular massage help you to reduce anxiety, increase sound sleep, and be active again? The only way to know if massage therapy can help your back pain is to schedule an appointment for your first session. If you are apprehensive about massage, read what Caroline, one of my back pain patients, told me about her first experience with massage therapy:

"When I went to my first appointment at a massage therapy center, I was impressed by how professional everyone was. The receptionist asked me to fill out a medical history form, and then one of the massage therapists took me in a room to take a short symptom history. She also gave me more information on massage and how it can help end back pain. I didn't realize the therapists were licensed after taking a two-year program and undergoing twenty-two hundred hours of practical training.

"After we chatted for about thirty minutes, another massage therapist, Greta, took me into a small room that was painted a very soothing blue. I remember there was classical music playing in the background, and aromatherapy candles were burning near the windowsill. Greta showed me to a dressing area where I exchanged my street clothes for a long white sheet, which I tucked discreetly around my body.

"At first, I sat on the long table, and Greta told me a bit about herself. She, too, was a young mother and had been a massage therapist for four years. I felt relieved that we could share parenting stories, and it eased my tension. Greta asked me to lie facedown on the table, and as I arranged the sheet around me, she dimmed the lights in the room. She then began to rub sweet-smelling sesame oil on my skin and softly kneaded my tightened muscles. Using a gentle, rocking motion, her hands worked up my back toward my shoulders and then down again. She paid special attention to painful trigger points, using her thumb and elbow to massage these areas. Sometimes I felt like her fingers were pointing right into my skin, but she said that's because my muscles were so tense. Greta focused mostly on my upper body—my neck, shoulders, and upper back—where my pain was the worst.

"After the massage, I was afraid to move. For the first time in weeks,

I was very relaxed and the back pain was almost nonexistent. As I got dressed, I realized that the range of motion in my arms was greater and the tension in my upper body was greatly reduced. I continued receiving 30-minute massages twice a week for six months. I attribute this complementary therapy to helping me heal completely from what was debilitating pain. I now have very little pain or stiffness, and I sleep soundly at night."

The options for complementing your *Pain-Free Back Program* with manual therapies are great. Start today, and get optimal relief from pain and stiffness.

Pain-Free Back Healing Touch Rx

- Review the various touch mechanisms as you decide on the type of bodywork that will be best for your back pain.
- Talk to your doctor about the various types of manual therapies to make sure massage will be healing and not hurtful.
- Ask your doctor for a referral to a licensed and experienced massage therapist.
- Make an appointment and evaluate how you feel during and after the massage therapy.
- If your doctor agrees, consider chiropractic or osteopathy for hands-on care for your back.
- Acupuncture may give you the extra boost necessary to alleviate nagging back pain. If you choose to try acupuncture, make sure the practitioner is experienced and uses sanitary procedures (disposable needles).

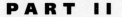

PART II

Special Situations

Making the Diagnosis

When forty-nine-year-old Vicki, a court stenographer, fell on her patio while trimming some of her plants, she thought she had simply bruised her lower back. "At first the back pain was excruciating. Then, after soaking in our outdoor Jacuzzi several times over the weekend and taking an over-the-counter pain medication, the pain eased some, and I thought my back was just bruised. I knew it was more serious when my back still hurt three weeks later, and I could hardly bend over."

After taking an X ray, Vicki was diagnosed with a fractured vertebra. I explained to Vicki that she had a lot of company, since there are about 750,000 new vertebral fractures in the Unites States each year. These fractures are usually caused by osteoporosis, or thinning of the bones, although they can also be the result of any trauma or, rarely, cancer. Osteoporosis is most common in women around or after menopause. Because Vicki had had a complete hysterectomy at age forty, we did a bone-density test. The test showed that her bones had become thin, which meant she would be at risk for more fractures in the future. I recommended that Vicki start the 6 steps in the *Pain-Free Back Program* to strengthen her bones and prevent future fractures.

While Vicki's fracture was extremely painful, as are 20 to 30 percent of vertebral fractures, most vertebral fractures may not be painful at the time they occur. It is not uncommon in older women to cite something as simple as raising a window or lifting a bag of groceries or a grandchild before a fracture occurs. Fractures cause sudden, severe back pain, felt deeply in an area in the back directly over the fracture. The pain is usually worse with any activity, and better with rest.

Diagnosing Your Back Pain

Getting an accurate diagnosis for your back pain will give you peace of mind that you're doing all you can to increase healing. During the examination, your doctor will assess the following:

- *Medical history.* Much of the information necessary for a correct diagnosis depends on how you describe your back pain: the location, severity, and what makes it feel better or worse. For example, is your pain in the upper or lower back? Does it radiate down your leg? Does it worsen after sitting for a period of time? Do you awaken at night with increased pain? The more specific you are in describing your pain, the more accurate your diagnosis and treatment will be.
- *Physical examination*
- *Imaging and laboratory tests*

Imaging Tests

The following imaging tests are commonly used to assess the causes of back and neck pain.

X Ray of the Spine

Your doctor might take an X ray of your back to help determine the cause of pain. An X ray can detect spinal fractures, infections, curvatures (scoliosis), tumors, bone spurs, and other changes in the bones of the spine. This commonly used test uses X ray electromagnetic energy beams to produce an image on film. Here are some examples of findings on X rays in a few common types of back pain:

Soft tissue pain. The X rays will appear normal if the cause of your back pain is soft tissue pain. Muscles, tendons, and ligaments do not usually show abnormalities on X rays. However, if you also have osteoarthritis or other problems that affect the bones and disk spaces, these will show on the X ray and will help your doctor to make a diagnosis.

Osteoarthritis. In osteoarthritis of the cervical, thoracic, or lumbar spine, X rays show narrowing of the cartilage disks between the vertebral bones and spurs along the spine.

Fibromyalgia. There are no X-ray changes in the spine with fibromyalgia syndrome; although doctors will look at these X rays to be certain no other problems are present to cause pain.

Ankylosing spondylitis. With this type of arthritis, the X rays will show changes in the sacroiliac joints in the lower back, which is where the pain usually starts. There may also be calcium bridges that have formed between the bones of the spine and later straightening of the spine.

Ruptured disk. Although X rays can show changes of osteoarthritis in the spine, which often accompany a ruptured disk, they do not show the actual nerves or whether there is pressure on a nerve because of the ruptured disc. Other imaging tests such as MRI, CT scan, or myelogram (see page 171) are needed to make this diagnosis.

Lumbar stenosis. X rays can show the osteoarthritis, which often accompanies lumbar stenosis, but other tests such as MRI or CT scan (see page 170) are needed to confirm this diagnosis.

Vertebral fracture. X ray of the spine can usually show a fracture in a vertebra. The bone is shortened or collapsed. This can affect more than one of the bones in the spine. It is the most common cause of the stooped-over posture found in some older women called a dowager's hump (see figure on page 170).

Magnetic Resonance Imaging (MRI)

MRI uses magnetism, radio waves, and a computer instead of radiation to gather accurate information about internal organs, structures, and tissues. This imaging technique is often used to evaluate all portions of the spine and can show abnormalities of cartilage and ligaments, as well as pressure on nerves from a ruptured disk, which routine X rays cannot show.

For patients with severe back pain, an MRI can reveal the cause. It can show a ruptured disk with more than 95 percent accuracy. An MRI can also show lumbar stenosis, which is a narrowing of the spinal canal that contains nerve roots. An MRI can detect other causes of back pain, including fractures, aortic aneurysm, infections in the spine, or cancer that affects the bones of the spine. Some people have feelings of claustrophobia because of the close situation in standard MRI equipment. You might feel more comfortable having this diagnostic test in an open MRI, or having your doctor give you a mild sedative before the test.

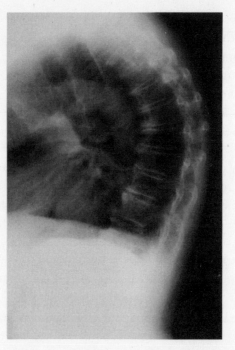

X ray of a Dowager's hump with osteoporosis

Computed Tomographic Scan (CT Scan)

A CT scan is a special computer-assisted X-ray procedure in which the X ray beam moves around the body, taking pictures from various angles. This imaging technique is used to give a more detailed diagnosis of the internal organs and is especially useful for imaging bones and organs in cases of severe back pain. The CT scan can detect a ruptured disk in more than 85 percent of cases in the lumbar spine and can occasionally suggest an abnormality when the disk is actually normal. CT is more accurate than X ray to find infection, fracture of a bone, or cancer. With an acceptable level of radiation exposure, a CT scan is done as an outpatient procedure and may be less confining than MRI for those who feel claustrophobic.

Bone Scan

A bone scan is used mainly when your doctor suspects something more than arthritis, such as an infection, cancer, or a fracture of a bone. It can detect abnormal areas of bone produced by these problems in all parts of the body's skeleton. The test is painless except for the injection of a small amount of radioactive dye followed in a few hours by a scan of the body while the patient lies on an X-ray table.

Bone-Density Test

A bone-density test checks for osteoporosis, thinning of the bones. If this test is positive, it can give early warning that you might be at risk for fractures in the spine, hip, wrist, or other bones—years before the fractures happen. The most common test used for an accurate diagnosis and follow-up of treatment is the DEXA test (dual energy X-ray absorptiometry) of the hip and lumbar spine. DEXA is easy, painless, and takes only a few minutes. The X-ray exposure is minimal, less than one-tenth of a chest X ray.

The heel sonogram is another common screening test. This test measures the bone density in the heel. You might see this test offered at malls and at health fairs. The heel sonogram takes three to four minutes and can help you decide whether you need to have the more specific DEXA test discussed above.

Myelogram

A myelogram requires an injection of dye into the spinal canal through a needle to show the rupture of a disk or other problems. Normally the dye would fill the spinal canal, as well as the nerve root sheaths, giving a revealing outline for an X ray. Yet, in an abnormal myelogram, there is an absence of dye in a specific area. This is called a "filling defect" and indicates that the nerve root or spinal cord is pinched or compressed. This test detects the ruptured disk.

The myelogram has more discomfort, requires an injection, and has a greater possibility of an unwanted side-effect such as a headache. Some experts now recommend an MRI of the lumbar spine. Then, if there is not a clear answer, a myelogram is performed. A CT scan may be combined with a myelogram to improve the accuracy of diagnosis, especially if a small piece of disk has broken off and is pressing on a nerve away from its root between the vertebrae.

Electromyelogram (EMG) and Nerve Conduction Study

These two tests are used in combination to diagnose sources of nerve or muscle pain. An electromyelogram (EMG) measures the activity of the muscles supplied by the nerves that are being irritated by your ruptured or herniated disc. A nerve conduction study tests the velocity in which the nerve transmits its signal. If the nerve is pinched, its ability to transmit a signal is reduced. Abnormal muscle activity and slowed nerve conduction may suggest a pinched or irritated nerve from a disk rupture.

Laboratory Tests

Specific laboratory blood tests might help your doctor decide the cause of your back pain, or eliminate certain causes of back pain from consideration. For example, if you have a ruptured disk, the blood tests will usually be normal. Some blood tests could suggest another problem such as arthritis or an infection causing your pain.

Screening Laboratory Tests
A complete blood count (CBC) measures the hemoglobin, red cells, white cells, and platelets and can find many of the common blood disorders, such as anemia, which can cause fatigue and tiredness. A screening test of blood chemistries can find abnormalities in liver, kidneys, or evidence of other internal organ problems.

Sedimentation Rate
The sedimentation rate (sed rate) measures how fast red blood cells fall to the bottom of a test tube. When inflammation is present, the blood's proteins clump together and become heavier than normal. The sedimentation rate can be high in inflammatory arthritis such as ankylosing spondylitis, infection, or other problems, but in osteoarthritis, soft tissue pain, and fibromyalgia the sed rate is usually normal.

Types of Back Pain

Not all back pain is the same. Just as the cause of pain varies, so will the treatment. For instance, osteoarthritis is a common cause of back pain and is treated with heat, exercise, and medications for pain and inflammation, among other therapies. While osteoporosis may cause similar pain to osteoarthritis, it is treated with medications to increase bone density and reduce fractures. Ruptured disk, yet another common cause of back pain, is treated with surgery in some cases. All of these problems cause pain— yet they all have effective but different treatments.

Soft Tissue Pain

Soft tissue pain, which comes from the muscles, tendons, and ligaments around the back, probably accounts for most cases of acute back pain. This back pain affects about half of all Americans each year. The exact causes are not known, and acute attacks of pain can happen even without unusual injury or strain—sometimes when we reach over to pick up a feather!

Signs and symptoms. Soft tissue pain is severe even if the underlying cause is not. Sometimes the pain is incapacitating. It can travel down a leg, just as true sciatica does, and for this reason is often called "sciatica." Many daily activities are limited by the pain, which usually improves within 7 to 10 days.

Soft tissue pain may combine with any other causes of back pain. If you don't find relief within 7 to 10 days, definitely check with your doctor to be sure no additional problems are causing the pain. It is common for these attacks of pain to flare a few times each year. They can happen in addition to osteoarthritis or other basic cause of back pain.

Diagnosis. Usually made after talking and examination and after other causes are eliminated.

Treatment. Moist heat, exercises, and medications, can relieve the pain much earlier and allow you to be active while you improve.

Osteoarthritis

Osteoarthritis can cause acute and chronic pain in the back and neck, depending on whether it attacks the lumbar spine or the cervical spine. This "wear-and-tear" type of arthritis is associated with aging and is especially common in those who have had previous neck or back injuries.

Signs and symptoms. The pain usually begins gradually, often many years after an injury, and becomes noticeable over a few months. At first, the arthritis pain is not severe, so you may ignore it. However, gradually the pain builds and begins to interfere with your activities. Initially, there may be stiffness and discomfort only after running or during other strenuous activity. Then, over a few years the pain and stiffness increases after walking, bending, and lifting. You may feel stiffness on arising in the morning that takes a few minutes to "work out" and stiffness after sitting in one position for a few minutes. Activities can continue with pain.

With osteoarthritis alone, the pain most commonly stays in the back, instead of traveling down the legs (sciatica). After a while, the stiffness becomes as limiting as the pain itself, making it harder to lean over to pick up your newspaper or tie your shoes. After months or even years of living with this nagging pain and limitation, or when activity becomes difficult or the pain interrupts sleep, most people decide to get medical help to relieve it.

Diagnosis. Blood tests can help eliminate other types of arthritis and other medical problems. X rays show changes of osteoarthritis in the spine. There may be narrowing of the cartilage of the disks of the spine but no destruction as in rheumatoid arthritis.

Treatment. The 6 steps in the *Pain-Free Back Program*, including stretching, strengthening, and aerobic or conditioning exercises, along with applications of moist heat, a prudent diet to lose weight or maintain a normal weight, lifestyle changes, and NSAIDs or other medications are treatment for osteoarthritis. Protecting your joints, as discussed on page 112, is important to avoid worsening of pain.

Common Risk Factors for Osteoarthritis

- Age (over forty-five)
- Overweight
- Athletics (wear-and-tear injuries)
- Changing forces (putting weight on one knee or hip)
- Gender (the chance of OA is the same for men and women between forty-five to fifty-five; after age fifty-five, OA is more common in women)
- Heavy, constant joint use
- Injury
- Joint injury by other types of arthritis
- Knee surgery
- Lack of exercise (weak muscles giving no support to aging joints)

Do You Have Osteoarthritis?

_____ Deep, aching pain in joints or the back
_____ Difficulty dressing or combing hair because of stiffness
_____ Difficulty gripping objects
_____ Difficulty sitting or bending over because of pain and stiffness
_____ Morning stiffness
_____ Pain in the back, hips, or knees when walking

_____ Stiffness after resting
_____ Swelling of joints such as the knees

Trigger Areas

Trigger areas may be present in the lower, middle, or upper back, or in the neck (see figure below). These small areas of soft tissue pain usually occur around muscles and are extremely tender when touched with slight pressure.

Signs and symptoms. Trigger areas are much more painful and tender than other areas of the back, even those nearby. Pressure on one of these trigger areas may also make you feel pain elsewhere (they trigger pain felt in other areas). For example, pressure on a trigger area in the upper back may cause pain that travels down one arm or up into the neck.

Diagnosis. After talking with and examination by your doctor of typical trigger points, and after eliminating other causes, a diagnosis is made.

Treatment. When trigger areas cause persistent, severe pain, your doctor can inject the areas with a local anesthetic and a small dose of a cortisone

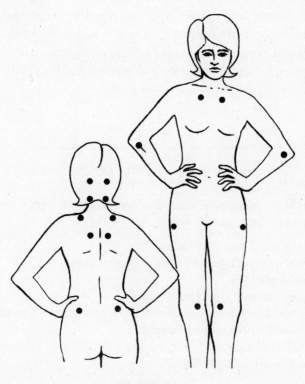

Trigger areas

medication (see page 201). Usually the painful trigger area and the "extra" pain areas are relieved by a single injection.

Osteoporosis

Osteoporosis is thinning of the bones. It is most common in women after the age of menopause or in men after age seventy. It is the most common cause of loss of height and stooped-over posture. It is also the most common cause of fractures in the spine and hip. The fractures can be painful and may limit your activity.

Signs and symptoms. There are no symptoms from osteoporosis because the bones become thin over years. If you do not discover the problem by a bone-density test, you may find it when you have a fracture in your wrist, spine, shoulder, or hip.

Diagnosis. The diagnosis is usually made after the first fracture when an X ray is taken. The diagnosis can be made much earlier by having a bone-density test. This test is recommended if you are at higher than normal risk for osteoporosis.

Treatment. Treatment includes finding any specific conditions contributing to osteoporosis, for example, smoking cigarettes, rheumatoid arthritis, or other medical problems. Then be sure you have a daily calcium intake of 1,500 mg (diet plus supplement) and supplemental vitamin D if your doctor advises. Add back exercises and gradually add walking, which are good natural stimulations for bone formation.

Common Risk Factors for Osteoporosis

Women after menopause, especially if not taking estrogen treatment and especially after age 65. Also:

- If you've had a fracture after age 40
- A family member with a fracture or osteoporosis
- Cigarette smoking
- Diseases such as rheumatoid arthritis
- Certain medications such as prednisone or other cortisone medications
- Underweight (thin for your height)
- Low calcium intake
- Inactive or sedentary lifestyle

Some of the Most Common Medications for Osteoporosis

Actonel (risedronate)
Fosamax (alendronate)
Evista (raloxifene)
Forteo (parathyroid hormone)
Miacalcin (calcitonin)

Add a medication to increase bone strength and reduce fractures. Your doctor will help you decide which of the medications is best for you. These can help lower the risk of fractures in the spine and hip by over 50 percent. And if you are unsteady or tend to fall, consider wearing hip protectors—a simple piece of clothing worn under your clothes, usually not noticeable—that lowers the risk of hip fracture by 50 percent if you happen to fall.

Fibromyalgia

When you have many areas of soft tissue pain in trigger areas that last for months, it might be fibromyalgia. Fibromyalgia can happen alone or along with other types of arthritis, such as osteoarthritis or rheumatoid arthritis.

Signs and symptoms. The pain is widespread over both sides of the body and includes the upper and lower areas of the back—pain everywhere. In fibromyalgia there are also typical locations for trigger areas in the neck, back, arms, and legs. Most people also feel fatigue that may be overwhelming. Other common problems in patients with fibromyalgia are difficulty sleeping at night, depression, and irritable bowel syndrome.

Diagnosis. Your doctor will make a diagnosis when the signs and symptoms above are present and other causes of back pain are excluded.

Treatment. Basic treatment for fibromyalgia is twice daily moist heat, and stretching and strengthening exercises. Once you can do the exercises starting on page 259, then gradually add aerobic or conditioning exercises such as walking, biking, swimming, or similar type of activity. Start with just one minute a day and slowly increase this time as you can do so without great pain.

Medications in fibromyalgia control pain and help to improve your ability to exercise. It might take trying a few different medications to find the ones that work best for your situation.

Possible Contributing Causes of Fibromyalgia

Decrease in serotonin (the chemical in the body associated with calming/anti-anxiety)

Aging

Female gender

High sensitivity to pain (even from normally nonpainful stimulation)

Inherited tendency

Magnesium deficiency

Menopause

Poor physical conditioning

Result of depression

Result of injury or accident

Sleep disorder

Stress

Surgery

Trauma to the nervous system

Common Symptoms of Fibromyalgia

Anxiety

Chronic headaches

Depression

Difficulty concentrating

Discoloration of hands and feet (Raynaud's disease) on exposure to cold

Dryness in mouth, nose or eyes

Fatigue

Irritable bowel syndrome

Morning stiffness

Pain

Painful menstrual cramps

Restless legs syndrome

Sleep problems

Swelling, numbness, and tingling in hands, arms, feet, and legs

Trigger areas

Urinary symptoms

Lumbar Disk Disease

The most common cause of true sciatica is a ruptured (herniated) disk in the lumbar spine.

Signs and symptoms. Back pain that travels down one leg, especially down the back of the leg, with burning or tingling, can be caused by pressure on the sciatic nerve as it leaves the spinal cord.

Diagnosis. The ruptured disk can be diagnosed by MRI, CT scan, or myelogram.

Treatment. A ruptured disk is treatable and the pain can be controlled without surgery in 90 percent of cases. Treatment includes moist heat and exercises (see Step 1). If no improvement, nerve blocks other pain

---

Warning Signs of Serious Problems in
Ruptured Lumbar and Cervical Disk—Call Your Doctor

Talk to your doctor if you have one or more of the following symptoms:

- Back or neck pain that worsens with coughing
- Back or neck pain that prevents sleep
- Difficulty controlling your bowels or bladder
- Weakness in one or both legs

---

treatments and evaluation for surgery are considered. However, in those cases where pain continues without relief or if muscles become weak, then surgery can relieve pressure on the nerve.

Cervical Disk Disease
Cervical disk disease is caused by pressure on a nerve in the cervical spine, most commonly from a ruptured disk.

Signs and symptoms. You might have neck pain with pain or numbness in one or both arms.

Diagnosis. The ruptured disk (or other problem) can be diagnosed by MRI, CT scan, or myelogram.

Treatment. Just as in the lumbar spine, most cases in the cervical spine get better without surgery. However, if the pain or numbness lasts more than seven days or if you find weakness in the muscles of an arm, see your doctor for a diagnosis.

Lumbar Stenosis
Lumbar stenosis, narrowing of the areas in the spine where nerves travel down the legs, is a common result of long-term osteoarthritis (see page 173). In addition to what you feel with the arthritis, this back pain travels down the legs when you walk because the activity causes swelling and pressure around the nerves.

Signs and symptoms. The back pain travels down both legs, and worsens after walking just a few blocks. When you stop walking, the pain in the legs also stops. After resting a few minutes, you may find that you can walk again until the pain comes back after a short period of time. Over time, usually months or a year, the distance you are able to walk shortens, causing you to walk less and less and to become less active. The pain may eventually become constant, even at rest, when it can also wake you at night.

Diagnosis. Lumbar stenosis is diagnosed by X rays and MRI or CT scan of the lumbar spine. It can be confused with leg pain from peripheral vascular disease (PVD), which is a blockage of the arteries in the legs. Your doctor can determine the cause of the pain with some simple tests of the arteries in the legs.

Treatment. To treat lumbar stenosis, continue the moist heat and exercises of Step 1) in the *Pain-Free Back Program.* If after two weeks you have little to no improvement, talk with your doctor about other available treatments, including nerve blocks for pain control and pain medication.

Many patients find improvement without surgery, but in this case if the pain doesn't improve, consider surgery evaluation. In many cases, an operation can remove pressure on the nerves, relieve pain, and allow you to walk without pain again.

Ankylosing Spondylitis

In ankylosing spondylitis, the joints and ligaments that allow the back to move become inflamed. The joints and bones become stiff and the back loses its flexibility. After years, the back can become completely stiff in one position. This type of arthritis pain in the lower back can start in the teens or early twenties and is more common in younger men.

Signs and symptoms. Ankylosing spondylitis pain starts gradually as a dull pain. It is often mistaken for an injury. Over time, the pain becomes more constant and may continue as mild or moderate pain. There is also usually stiffness on arising in the morning or stiffness after sitting for a few minutes, along with fatigue.

There are other serious problems with this type of arthritis. Stiffness starting in the lower back may gradually work its way up to the neck over a period of five to ten years. It might also stop at any point in the back. About half of those with ankylosing spondylitis experience pain, stiffness, or swelling in other joints such as the hips or shoulders.

Diagnosis. Your doctor can make a diagnosis by physical examination and X rays of the spine. Most patients with this arthritis and back pain have a positive blood test for HLA-B27 antigen, an inherited protein that increases the chances for ankylosing spondylitis.

Treatment. Use moist heat, exercises to stretch and strengthen the back, and anti-inflammatory medications. Exercises are extremely important to help prevent deformity, especially a stooped-over deformity of the back. Even if the back becomes stiff, you can still be active if you avoid a stooped-over posture. If there is not enough improvement to allow good pain control and activity, one of the biologic medications used to treat rheumatoid arthritis can be added. These new drugs usually give a quick response, a greater chance of remission of the arthritis pain and swelling, and a higher chance of stopping any permanent damage.

Biologic Disease-Modifying Drugs (DMARDs)

Brand Name	Generic Name
Enbrel	etanercept
Kineret	anakinra
Remicade	infliximab
Humira	adalimumab

Back Arthritis with Other Problems

Arthritis with pain and stiffness similar to ankylosing spondylitis can happen in persons with psoriasis, ulcerative colitis, Crohn's disease or other medical problems. The diagnosis is made by your doctor based on examination and X rays. Treatments are similar to those used for ankylosing spondylitis, in addition to specific treatment of the other underlying problem. Exercises are an important part of the treatment for all types of back pain.

Other Medical Problems Associated with Back Pain

Because back pain might be an indication of a serious problem, do not assume your pain is caused by any of the conditions mentioned in this section until you've spoken with your doctor. Back pain might also indicate:

- Infection in or around the bones of the spine
- Aneurysm (enlargement) of the aorta
- Kidney stone
- Disease in an internal organ in the abdomen
- Cancer of a bone in the spine

Combination Problems

If your back pain has worsened or the medications that once worked now don't help at all, you may be dealing with more than one cause of back pain. This is a very common problem, yet it can lead to frustration and more pain as the first known cause is treated, but other untreated causes still create pain. For example, you might have osteoarthritis of the spine and still develop other painful conditions in the back such as ruptured disk, pain from muscles and tendons, scoliosis (curvature), or another medical problem. Or, if you have fibromyalgia and worsening of lower back pain, another problem may have developed, such as osteoarthritis or osteoporosis with spinal fracture.

Anytime your back pain changes, especially if it is more painful, it is a good idea to check with your doctor. Some serious medical problems such as infections, kidney stones, aortic aneurysm (enlargement of the aorta in the abdomen), or less common causes such as cancer can cause back pain. Each cause has specific and effective treatment, so getting an accurate diagnosis is vital.

Here are some suggestions for some common combinations of back pain to consider when your back pain changes its course.

INITIAL DIAGNOSIS: OSTEOARTHRITIS
COMBINATION PROBLEM: PAINFUL TRIGGER AREA

If your diagnosis is osteoarthritis in the spine causing back or neck pain and the pain takes a more severe turn, it may be more than just osteo-arthritis. One of the most common second causes is pain in muscles and tendons around the spine (soft tissue pain). The exact cause is not known, but this pain may come on suddenly with or without any unusual activity or strain. It may be even more severe than the original arthritis pain. It can prevent sleep and make every movement during your day painful. There are often one or two small areas in the back or neck that are especially painful to touch and the pain may travel down one leg or one arm when the painful area is touched, as if there were a ruptured disk.

These trigger areas are extremely painful, but they are not a dangerous cause of pain by themselves. If no other problems are present, they can be treated with moist heat, warm shower, and exercises. If they don't improve, a local injection by your doctor may give quick relief.

INITIAL DIAGNOSIS: OSTEOARTHRITIS
COMBINATION PROBLEM: SPINAL FRACTURE FROM OSTEOPOROSIS

If you have a diagnosis of osteoarthritis in the lower back and your pain suddenly becomes worse, especially after you lift something, raise a window, or fall, you might have a spinal compression fracture, which is most commonly due to osteoporosis. This pain usually improves in days with pain medication and avoiding positions of pain (usually resting in a position about halfway between sitting and lying flat is the most comfortable).

In this case, your doctor can make a quick diagnosis with an X ray and other tests, and you can start simple treatment to prevent more fractures in the future. There may even be other causes of the osteoporosis that need to be discovered and treated.

INITIAL DIAGNOSIS: OSTEOARTHRITIS
COMBINATION PROBLEM: RUPTURED DISK

If you suffer from back pain due to osteoarthritis in the spine but pain becomes severe and travels down one leg, you might also have a ruptured disk. The sensation might feel like hot water running down your leg. You might also feel numbness and tingling in that leg. If the pain prevents sleep, if it hurts when you cough, or if your bowel or bladder habits change, then see your doctor right away. Ruptured disks usually improve over a few weeks with moist heat, rest, exercise, and medications. The large majority of cases will not need surgery.

INITIAL DIAGNOSIS: OSTEOARTHRITIS
COMBINATION PROBLEM: LUMBAR STENOSIS

The wear-and-tear of osteoarthritis on the lumbar spine can gradually lead to narrowing and pressure on nerves as they leave the spinal cord and travel down the legs. In some cases, instead of a single area of pressure on one nerve as in a ruptured disk, there is a less localized area of narrowing. This can cause pain in the back and legs when you walk. There may be little or no pain in the lower back at rest but pain in the legs when walking that goes away when you stop and rest for a few minutes.

As it worsens, the distance before the pain becomes severe gets shorter and shorter. Circulation problems in the legs (peripheral vascular disease) can cause similar feelings, but your doctor can order easy, nonpainful tests to tell if the circulation is normal. The lumbar spine MRI can show lumbar stenosis and make the diagnosis.

The treatment for lumbar stenosis is like the treatment for osteoarthritis in the spine—moist heat, exercises for the back, and medications. But if there is no relief (walking does not get less painful), then surgery can offer good relief in some cases. A neurosurgeon or orthopedic surgeon can tell you your options and chances of success.

INITIAL DIAGNOSIS: FIBROMYALGIA
COMBINATION PROBLEM: PAINFUL TRIGGER AREAS

Fibromyalgia causes pain almost everywhere, but if the back or neck pain becomes suddenly severe and seems to be from a small area of tenderness, this trigger area can be treated with moist heat, warm shower, and if severe may be controlled with a local injection by your doctor. The typical trigger area is localized and causes pain that may be felt in other areas when it is touched with only mild pressure.

These single trigger areas are best treated by moist heat (warm shower, moist towel, or similar) and exercises—even though you may need to do fewer repetitions for a few days. If still not improved, an injection by your doctor of a local anesthetic plus cortisone derivative usually gives relief.

INITIAL DIAGNOSIS: FIBROMYALGIA
COMBINATION PROBLEM: OSTEOARTHRITIS

If you suffer from fibromyalgia and have worsening of lower back pain, another problem may have developed such as osteoarthritis in the spine. This wear-and-tear problem causes pain gradually, with stiffness when you wake up in the morning and stiffness after sitting. It can cause pain on walking and standing.

A good treatment in this situation is moist heat such as a warm shower, exercises and a nonsteroidal anti-inflammatory drug (NSAID). One of the complementary treatments, discussed on page 78, may help. If it's too painful to do the exercises, then check with your doctor to be sure no other problems are present.

INITIAL DIAGNOSIS: FIBROMYALGIA
COMBINATION PROBLEM: SPINAL FRACTURE

Sudden back pain, especially after lifting, may be the sign of a compression fracture in the spine in addition to your fibromyalgia. This is caused by osteoporosis, is treated with moist heat, warm shower, rest (halfway between lying and sitting), and pain medications. Excellent treatment is available for osteoporosis to prevent future fractures.

INITIAL DIAGNOSIS: FIBROMYALGIA

COMBINATION PROBLEM: RUPTURED DISK

When the pain of fibromyalgia changes or becomes worse in one area, such as one leg or one arm, it is possible that there is pressure on a nerve from a disk (described above). If the pain travels down an arm, or there is numbness, tingling, or weakness in an arm, this suggests a problem combined with fibromylagia. If the problem persists, an MRI of the cervical spine (if the pain is in an arm) or the lumbar spine (if the pain is in a leg) can help sort out these problems. The MRI can show if there is pressure on a nerve from a ruptured disk.

Medications and
Surgery for Back Pain

While many people believe that a pill will solve their back problems indefinitely, medications alone are *not* the answer to ending back pain. Yes, it is true that in most cases medications can help to control pain, which will allow you to start your exercises. As you read in Step 1, the more you move around and begin to strengthen your muscles with exercise, the faster your back pain will resolve. Medications, in combination with the *Pain-Free Back Program* steps, can make it easier to return to other areas of your life that back pain has taken away. Nevertheless, depending on medications alone to protect your back from further injury and pain is not realistic.

That's why it's helpful to think about medications as *one part* of your *Pain-Free Back Program*. Don't expect medications to solve your back problem. However, do expect them to help control pain while the 6-step *Pain-Free Back Program* begins to work. If the medications you're taking for back pain don't give you full relief, you may not be taking the most effective medications available. For example, Julia tried five nonsteroidal anti-inflammatory drugs (NSAIDs) before finding one that worked to resolve her back pain caused by a herniated disk. She finally found relief with an over-the-counter medication, taking it several times through the course of a day. Alternatively, Richard suffers with osteoarthritis in the spine. Once this was diagnosed, he immediately started on a COX-2 NSAID, a prescription anti-inflammatory medication, and his osteoarthritis pain was alleviated within a few days.

We know that every case of back pain is different. You need to know in advance that your doctor cannot know the exact medication that will work best to eliminate your pain or back problem. It usually takes a trial of a few different medications to find pain relief. In addition, it often requires more than one medication to achieve your goal of pain relief. The good news is that if you are patient, there are so many excellent medications available that you will eventually find the combination that gives you sufficient relief.

To find the best medications as quickly as possible, it helps to understand how they are used by your doctor. Rather than using a random approach, hoping that some medication works, your doctor should have a plan that will allow pain relief, starting with the lowest doses, the least expense, and the most effective results.

Rate Your Pain

Before I discuss the countless medications used to treat back pain, I'd like you to rate your pain, using the chart below, and share this information with your physician. According to your response, your doctor can determine if you should stay on the same medication, try a different medication, or consider a combination of medications.

Chart Your Relief after Medication

Review the chart and rate your pain after medication with 0 meaning no pain at all, and 10 being the worst pain imaginable. For instance, if you charted your pain before medicine as an 8 or 9 and then it comes down to a 3 or 4 after taking the medication, you might have found a combination that is useful for pain control. In contrast, if your pain level is a 1 or 2 and then soars to a 9 or 10, your doctor needs to evaluate you to find out if a new problem might be causing the pain.

Eventually, you'll find a level of pain control (around 3 to 5 for most people) that is livable and allows you to continue the strengthening exercises to protect back from further injury and pain.

Pain Rating Scale

0	1	2	3	4	5	6	7	8	9	10

No Pain   Livable Pain   Worst Pain

Use the BPI to Assess Your Daily Pain

Now use the following 10-question pain assessment (I call it a Back Pain Index or BPI) to rate your pain on a daily basis. This will let you and your doctor know if the back pain is improving, the same, or worsening. You may need a change of medication, or there may be another reason for the pain.

Back Pain Index (BPI)

Circle a number that reflects how your back pain interferes with each of the following 10 lifestyle areas:

0 = No Problem   10 = Major Difficulty

1. Personal care (bathing, styling hair, dressing, etc.)
   0   1   2   3   4   5   6   7   8   9   10

2. Daily household responsibilities
   0   1   2   3   4   5   6   7   8   9   10

3. Work
   0   1   2   3   4   5   6   7   8   9   10

4. Sleep
   0   1   2   3   4   5   6   7   8   9   10

5. Relationships
   0   1   2   3   4   5   6   7   8   9   10

6. Pain-Free Back exercises
   0   1   2   3   4   5   6   7   8   9   10

7. Sexual activities
   0   1   2   3   4   5   6   7   8   9   10

8. Sports and recreational activities
   0   1   2   3   4   5   6   7   8   9   10

9. Outlook on life/disposition
   0   1   2   3   4   5   6   7   8   9   10

10. Hobbies
    0   1   2   3   4   5   6   7   8   9   10

Calculate Your BPI: Add together all the numbers circled and divide by 10. The resulting quotient is your Back Pain Index. Figure out your BPI each day for two weeks, and keep track of this number. If your score decreases (i.e., goes from 8 to 4), that's a sign that your back pain is improving and that the 6-step *Pain-Free Back Program* is working. If the score increases (i.e., goes from 3 to 8), talk to your doctor. You may need to review the 6-step program again to ensure you're following all the suggestions correctly, or consider that a different medication might be necessary to give you optimal relief and a greater quality of life.

Over-the-Counter Pain Medications

Before you opt for powerful prescription pain medications, make sure you've tried over-the-counter pain medications that are available at many supermarkets and pharmacies. These analgesics (pain relievers) and NSAIDs are widely advertised and are proven to give relief in many cases. And even if these pain relievers don't work well, the information will help your doctor decide which medication to prescribe next. Moreover, over-the-counter pain relievers might be able to improve your pain when used alone or later as an occasional supplement to other prescribed medications.

These medications are usually safe when taken according to the directions on the label, but check with your doctor's office to be sure over-the-counter pain medications are safe for you and that you take the right dose. If you have heart disease, liver disease, kidney disease, or peptic ulcers, definitely check with your doctor before taking the medication.

Commonly Used Over-the-Counter Pain Medications

Brand Name	Generic Name
Anacin	aspirin (with caffeine)
Advil	ibuprofen
Aleve	naproxen
Ascriptin, Bufferin	buffered aspirin
Bayer and other brands	aspirin
Ecotrin	enteric-coated aspirin
Excedrin Extra Strength	aspirin
Motrin	ibuprofen
Panex	acetaminophen
Tylenol	acetaminophen

Aspirin (Excedrin, Bayer, Anacin, Ecotrin)

Aspirin products are the oldest over-the-counter pain medication. In low doses, aspirin helps control mild to moderate pain. In higher doses, aspirin can cause upset stomach, peptic ulcers and bleeding, ringing in the ears (tinnitus), and other problems. Aspirin can increase bruising, especially over the arms. If your doctor has recommended aspirin (only in low dose) to protect the heart and blood vessels, it can be taken along with a prescription NSAID. However, you should not take any higher doses of aspirin products if you are taking a prescription NSAID.

Aspirin products should not be used if you are taking warfarin (Coumadin). Aspirin is often combined with another medication to increase pain relief.

Acetaminophen (Tylenol, Panex)

Acetaminophen can relieve mild to moderate pain. It should start to give relief within an hour and can be taken as often as the directions on the label allow. Acetaminophen is not likely to cause upset stomach or intestinal bleeding and can even be taken while you are taking most other medications, including blood thinners such as warfarin (Coumadin). Acetaminophen can also be taken as a supplement to help breakthrough pain when you are taking most other arthritis medications.

If you have liver disease or kidney disease, check with your doctor to be sure you know how much acetaminophen you should take.

Over-the-Counter NSAIDs (Advil, Motrin, Aleve)

You might try an over-the-counter nonsteroidal anti-inflammatory medication to ease back pain. These medications reduce inflammation caused by injury, muscle aches, or arthritis. In fact, some prescription NSAID medications are available in lower doses over-the-counter. These doses can be used to relieve pain, if acetaminophen (Tylenol) doesn't give enough relief.

If you follow the directions on the label, over-the-counter NSAIDs usually do not have serious side effects. But if you take extra doses, you may be at risk for abdominal pain, peptic ulcer, bleeding, and other problems, just the same as with the prescription doses of these medications.

If you have heart disease, peptic ulcers, kidney disease, or liver disease check with your doctor before you try one of these medications. If one is safe for you to try, you can take it as needed for pain as often as the label directions allow. If you develop upset stomach, abdominal pain, or another new problem, then stop the medication until you check with your doctor's office. These medications should not be used if you are taking warfarin (Coumadin).

Prescription Pain Relievers

When over-the-counter medications do not resolve your back pain, talk to your doctor about prescribing a stronger pain medication. The following represent the most commonly used prescriptions for back pain.

**Prescription Nonsteroidal
Anti-Inflammatory Drugs (NSAIDs)**

If over-the-counter medications don't work well enough, your doctor may prescribe an NSAID. These may include higher doses of the over-the-counter medications, or they might include other medications that give the effect of high doses of over-the-counter medications but with fewer side effects. For example, aspirin in full doses (12 to 16 tablets over a 24-hour period) can be quite effective for calming inflammation and ending pain. Yet, aspirin in large doses increases the risk of peptic ulcers and bleeding more than other available medications.

There are two types of NSAIDs available: traditional NSAIDs and COX-2 NSAIDs.

Traditional NSAIDs. Each of the traditional NSAIDs is effective for pain and inflammation (see chart on page 192). With just one or a few tablets daily, these traditional NSAIDs have fewer side effects than high doses of aspirin. Your doctor will choose one of this group based on your back pain, taking into account other medical problems, the cost of the drug, and even your insurance coverage. There are over twenty choices, and most people find one that gives good relief from pain and inflammation without side effects. If you find that after weeks, months, or years your NSAID loses its effect on your pain, it may be helpful to try one of the others (which may be one reason there are so many available). When you take a traditional NSAID regularly, you should check your blood pressure and have blood tests for kidney, liver, and complete blood count every three to four months.

Prescription NSAIDs must be used carefully in patients with heart disease, kidney disease, hypertension, or if you have had peptic ulcers. Traditional NSAIDs are not taken with blood thinners such as warfarin (Coumadin) because they might increase risk of bleeding. About 2 to 3 percent of those who take these drugs regularly have a chance of peptic ulcer and bleeding each year. The highest risk of gastrointestinal bleeding is in those persons who

- Are over age sixty-five
- Have already had a peptic ulcer
- Are taking aspirin or prednisone
- Are taking warfarin (Coumadin)
- Have other serious medical problems

If you are at higher risk for peptic ulcer and bleeding, your doctor may add another medication to prevent peptic ulcer and decrease this risk (see page 193). Always take your traditional NSAID with food to avoid stomach upset.

Your doctor will tell you when your traditional NSAIDs should be stopped before having surgery since they can increase bleeding. When you take one of these regularly, don't forget blood tests every few months, especially tests for kidney function (BUN and creatinine), and a complete blood count.

Some Commonly Used Traditional NSAIDS

Brand Name	Generic Name
Ansaid	flurbiprofen
Arthrotec	diclofenac plus misoprostol
Clinoril	sulindac
Daypro	oxaprozin
Disalcid, Mono-Gesic	salsalate
Dolobid	diflunisal
Feldene	piroxicam
Indocin	indomethacin
Lodine	etodolac
Meclomen	meclofenamate
Motrin	ibuprofen
Nalfon	fenoprofen
Naprelan	naproxen
Naprosyn	naproxen
Orudis, Oruvail	ketoprofen
Relafen	nabumetone
Tolectin	tolmetin
Trilisate	choline magnesium trisalicylate
Voltaren	diclofenac
Zorprin	aspirin

Common Side Effects of NSAIDs

Abdominal pain
Abnormal liver tests (blood tests)
Asthma in those allergic
Bruising or bleeding more easily

Can aggravate or cause kidney (renal) failure

Diminished effect of diuretics

Dizziness

Gastritis

Heartburn

Increased blood pressure (hypertension)

Indigestion

Intestinal bleeding

Lower hemoglobin (anemia)

May affect other medications taken

May decrease platelet effect (can affect bleeding)

May change the effect of other medication, such as oral diabetic medications, warfarin (Coumadin), beta-blockers, ACE inhibitors, diuretics

Peptic ulcer

Ringing in the ears (tinnitus)

Sodium retention and edema in the feet and legs

Commonly Used H2 Blockers

Brand Name	Generic Name
Axid	nizatidine
Pepcid	famotidine
Tagamet	cimetidine
Zantac	ranitidine

These medications are used to lower the chance of upset stomach from NSAIDs or other medications. They are also used to treat and prevent peptic ulcer disease. However, taking one of these medications has not been shown to prevent the risk of bleeding from peptic ulcers when you take one of the traditional NSAIDs. To lower the risk of bleeding, you must take Cytotec (misoprostol), one of the PPI (Proton Pump Inhibitor) drugs, or one of the COX-2 NSAIDs.

Commonly Used Proton Pump Inhibitor (PPI) Medications

Brand Name	Generic Name
Aciphex	rabeprazole
Nexium	esomeprazole

Commonly Used PPI Medications *(continued)*

Brand Name	Generic Name
Prevacid	lansoprazole
Prilosec	omeprazole
Protonix	pantoprazole

COX-2 NSAIDS. The second type of nonsteroidal anti-inflammatory drugs available are the COX-2 NSAIDs. These provide effective treatment for pain and inflammation and are currently recommended over the traditional NSAIDs for use in arthritis pain by the American Pain Society because of their effectiveness and safety.

COX-2 NSAIDs have about the same success rate as the traditional NSAIDs for treatment of inflammation, pain and stiffness in many types of arthritis. However, the NSAIDs may also give relief from other types of pain *not* related to arthritis, including dental and surgical pain. Because COX-2 NSAIDs can relieve pain other than arthritis pain, they are beneficial in treating back pain that might have various causes.

The COX-2 NSAIDs greatly reduce the chance of peptic ulcer disease and bleeding, so they are safer for regular use if they give relief of your back pain. When taking a COX-2 NSAID, it is not routine to add a medication to protect from peptic ulcer disease. And you do not need to stop taking the COX-2 NSAID before having surgery because there is no increased chance of bleeding. A COX-2 NSAID can be taken with a blood thinner such as warfarin (Coumadin), with continued monitoring.

As with traditional NSAIDs, COX-2 NSAIDs should be used with caution if you have heart disease, kidney disease, or hypertension. While taking one of these medications, it's a good idea to check blood tests, especially kidney function tests (BUN and creatinine) and get a complete blood count every three to four months for safety.

COX-2 NSAIDs

Brand Name	Generic Name
Bextra	valdecoxib
Celebrex	celecoxib
Mobic	meloxicam
Vioxx	rofecoxib

Mixing Supplements and Meds

Always talk to your doctor before taking any medication—over-the-counter or prescription—with dietary supplements, including your daily vitamins, minerals, or botanicals. Some supplements, particularly herbs like ginkgo, which thins the blood, may cause excessive bleeding when combined with aspirin or an NSAID.

Words of Caution

Did you know that . . .

- Stomach bleeding caused by NSAIDs is the most common serious drug reaction, resulting in over 16,500 deaths and over 107,000 hospitalizations annually in the United States?
- Most people who have NSAID-related stomach bleeding have no warning signs?
- If you are over sixty-five, have a history of ulcers, or take steroids or blood thinners, you are at highest risk for NSAID-related stomach problems?
- Because alcohol irritates the stomach lining, drinking it while taking over-the-counter NSAIDs can increase your risk of peptic ulcer and bleeding?
- Combining cold medications with over-the-counter pain medications can be toxic, especially if the cold medication also contains a pain-killer such as aspirin?
- Taking acetaminophen with alcohol, even moderate amounts, may increase the risk of liver problems?
- Using an NSAID during pregnancy may cause damage to the unborn child?

Cortisone-Type Drugs

Cortisone derivatives are most commonly used in back pain as injections. A small dose of cortisone derivative combined with a local anesthetic can give quick relief in soft tissue pain and trigger areas. Injecting a low dose is safer than giving larger doses by mouth, which can affect the entire body. Cortisone injections are also used for relief of chronic back pain in nerve blocks, as discussed on page 201.

Occasionally, prednisone or another cortisone derivative may be given by mouth for a short period of time to help decrease inflammation when there is a ruptured disk with sciatica and severe pain.

Low doses of prednisone may be used at times when there is inflammation in the back from ankylosing spondylitis or related arthritis. In these cases, the lowest possible dose is used for the shortest time needed.

Commonly Used Corticosteroid Medications

Brand Name	Generic Name
Aristocort	triamcinolone
Celestone	betamethasone
Decadron, Hexadrol, Kenalog	dexamethasone
Deltasone, Sterapred, Metacortin, Orasone	prednisone
Medrol, Depo Medrol	methylprednisolone
Prelone, Orapred	prednisolone

Muscle Relaxants

When back or neck pain is from a muscle spasm, a muscle relaxant can usually give relief. It may be hard to tell if some or all of your pain is actually coming from muscle spasm and tightness. Many times in these cases, one of the back muscles is hard to touch and is noticeably tight and swollen. Your doctor may try one of these medications to see its effect. If there is major improvement, these can be continued. As the underlying problem is treated and improves, muscle relaxants are usually not necessary for long-term treatment.

Commonly Used Muscle Relaxants

Brand Name	Generic Name
Flexeril	cyclobenzaprine
Parafon Forte	chlorzoxazone
Robaxin	methocarbamol
Skelaxin	metaxalone
Soma	carisopodol
Valium	diazepam
Zanaflex	tizanidine

Opioid (Narcotic) Analgesics

When other medications fail to give you pain relief and if you're experiencing severe limitation in activity and function, narcotic medications may be prescribed. These opioid analgesics are now accepted for use in severe back pain. Many patients find that these medications give excellent pain relief and allow a return to near normal activity. The side effects of these drugs are well-known and usually can be managed.

Until the past few years, narcotic analgesics have had limited use because of the fear of addiction. Although there is a physical tolerance (dependence) when these drugs are taken on a regular basis, true drug addiction (the need to continue even when the drug is harmful) is actually quite uncommon. Those who have had problems with drug abuse seem to be at most risk for developing addiction to narcotics prescribed for back pain, so careful monitoring is necessary in those cases. Whenever these medications are used, your doctor will likely require closer supervision and follow-up, since these are controlled drugs and have the potential for abuse. In our clinic, we require that patients who continue to use these medications find pain relief and are able to increase their activity, function, and exercise.

For relief of chronic back pain, several long-acting types of opioid (narcotic) analgesics are available that give a sustained level of relief over 12 to 72 hours. This is preferable to short-acting forms of narcotics that must be taken more frequently and often give incomplete or irregular relief of pain.

Tramadol is a pain medication that is included in this category because it is a weak opioid (narcotic) analgesic. Although tramadol may cause nausea or mild sedation, the symptoms are usually not severe.

A common side effect of opioid (narcotic) analgesics is constipation, which usually can be managed easily with mild laxatives and diet. Some of the other most common side effects of the opioid (narcotic) analgesics are listed.

Commonly Used Opioid (Narcotic) Analgesics

Generic Name	Common Brand Name
codeine	Combined with acetaminophen (Tylenol #3)
hydrocodone	Combined with acetaminophen (Vicodin, Lortab, Lorcet)
	Combined with ibuprofen (Vicoprofen)
	Combined with aspirin (Lortab ASA)

Commonly Used Opioid (Narcotic) Analgesics *(continued)*

Generic Name	Common Brand Name
hydromorphone	Dilaudid
meperidine	Demerol
morphine	MSIR, others
oxycodone	with acetaminophen (Tylox, Percocet)
propoxyphene	Darvon; combined with acetaminophen (Darvocet)

Long-Acting Narcotics for Chronic Back Pain

Oxycontin (oxycodone)
MS-Contin, Kadian (morphine controlled release)
Duragesic (fentanyl, transdermal) patch

Common Side Effects of Opioid (Narcotic) Analgesics

Constipation
Decreased concentration
Physical withdrawal after regular use
Sedation
Sexual dysfunction
Sweating

Supplemental Analgesics

Some medications (supplemental analgesics) were originally developed as antidepressants, but over the years have been shown to help give relief for back pain and other types of pain. For instance, tricyclic antidepressants have been proven to relieve pain in some patients, but these medications are not typical analgesics and do not have the side effects of some analgesics. They are commonly used in back pain from fibromyalgia; pain from injuries; pain in muscles, tendons, and ligaments; and pain from osteoarthritis.

Because the doses of these supplemental analgesics when used for pain are much lower than when used for depression, the side effects are also much lower. In fact, most patients tolerate these medications well if they happen to get pain relief.

A number of other supplemental pain medicines were developed originally for other purposes, such as seizure disorders. Your doctor can help you decide if one of these less commonly prescribed medications might be used in your case.

Commonly Used Tricyclic Antidepressants

Brand Name	Generic Name
Elavil	amitriptyline
Norpramin	desipramine
Pamelor	nortriptyline
Sinequan	doxepin
Tofranil	imipramine

Common Side Effects of Tricyclic Antidepressants

Sedation—sleepiness (this is positive if it aids in sleep at night)
Constipation
Mouth dryness
Less need to urinate (might may be helpful for those with an overactive bladder, but check with your doctor if this happens)
Dizziness
Problems with memory, concentration, or confusion
Heart rhythm abnormalities (uncommon except at high doses)
Sweating

Treating Depression

If your back pain becomes chronic (lasts longer than three months), you may become depressed as the cycle of pain leads to less activity and even more pain (see page 5). It's helpful to recognize depression early and accept it as a one part of your pain problem. (Depression and back pain is discussed on page 130.)

Excellent treatment is available using medications and psychological counseling. A psychiatrist or psychologist is skilled at successfully treating this problem and helping you to understand how pain influences your mind, body, and emotions.

Most people find that as depression improves, daily activity increases, which will help your overall pain and function improve.

Medications for Sleep

If pain is preventing your sleep, then effective pain relief is the answer to a restful night's sleep. If depression is causing restless sleep, then treatment of your depression will be the most effective treatment of your sleep problem.

If you and your doctor feel that your lack of restful sleep is a separate problem and warrants treatment, there are several good options. A natural treatment such as the botanical valerian or passionflower might be helpful. Many of my patients feel relaxed after drinking a soothing cup of chamomile tea before bedtime. Others find over-the-counter melatonin, a supplement, to be helpful in resetting your biological clock to allow a return to your usual sleep pattern. Melatonin may also cause you to feel sleepy the next day, so use with caution.

Other medications are available by prescription to help sleep. Discuss the problem with your doctor and consider a trial of one of these to see if improvement in sleep might help back pain, stiffness, and energy. The short-acting medications are preferred so you are not groggy in the morning. You may find that occasional use of one of the medications can help you maintain restful sleep.

Sleep Medications

Brand Name	Generic Name
Ambien	zolpidem
Sonata	zaleplon
Restoril	temazepam

Other Medical Treatments for Back Pain

For back pain that is difficult to control, it's important to find ways to make the pain "livable." Pain management techniques are available now that allow pain relief and increase in activity. Some treatments that might be used include:

- Local injections in painful trigger areas in the back
- Injections to temporarily or more permanently block painful nerves
- Nerve stimulation with TENS (transcutaneous electrical nerve stimulation), discussed on page 161.

- Surgery to implant a pump for longer-term or continuous morphine pain control
- Surgery to implant electrical nerve stimulators

Injections

When conservative treatment fails to relieve back pain, an injection in the painful area in and around the spine may give relief. There are several types of injections and sites to inject, depending on the cause of pain. Usually a cortisone derivative is used for the injection. This can be given with or without a local anesthetic.

Your doctor may inject the epidural space (around the spinal cord), the facet joints (near the vertebral body), or the general soft tissue area around the spine (such as muscles) with the goal of decreasing inflammation and pain.

Many patients benefit from injections for pain relief, including:

- Those with severe, disabling back pain who do not choose to have open, traditional surgery on the spine
- Those who are too high risk for surgery because of medical conditions such as heart or lung disease
- Those who are frail and elderly
- Those who have had previous back surgery with recurrent pain, resulting from scarring or inflammation remaining around the area
- Those with persistent sciatica after conservative treatment

Many back pain patients find reduced stiffness in the lower back immediately after an injection, including improved exercise tolerance, or decreased muscle spasm in the back. One study of injections even showed an improvement in overall energy and quality of life in selected patients.

If you have any neurological deficits, such as weakness or abnormal sensation in either or both legs, then injections are probably not the answer for you. And, as with other medications, the best outcome for this procedure occurs only when it is used in combination with back strengthening and flexibility exercises, physical therapy, and the other steps in this program.

Following are commonly used injection procedures for back pain:

Epidural injection. This involves injecting a steroid into the space around the spinal cord (epidural space). In the hands of an experienced pain physician, this may help subacute or chronic lower back pain by decreasing local inflammation. While more than one injection may be helpful, this area should not be injected more than three times at the same site, with each injection being at least one month apart.

Facet joint injection. This procedure involves injecting a steroid with or without a local anesthetic into a facet joint, one of the small joints around the spine. It can be beneficial in some cases of degenerative joint disease or in osteoarthritis of the lumbar spine. The decision to use an injection is made after it has been decided that your back pain is coming in part from the facet joints. An imaging test such as CT or MRI may help make this decision.

Local injection. The surrounding ligaments and soft tissues around the spine can be the source of inflammatory pain in some instances. Injecting a steroid with or without a local anesthetic in this area can be safe and effective in pain relief, decreasing inflammation in many cases.

Chymopapain injection. One alternative for treating pain from a herniated disk is with the injection of an enzyme (chymopapain) into the center of the intervertebral disk (called chemonucleolysis or CNL). Although the procedure is rarely performed in the United States, it is less invasive than surgery. The enzyme is a common ingredient in meat tenderizers and is meant to soften and degrade (break down) the disk itself, thus shrinking it. The goal is to relieve pressure on the sciatic nerve. The procedure may take just a few minutes, but complete pain relief might take days or even months. CNL is found to be as helpful in relieving sciatic pain as laminectomy, a surgical procedure (described on page 206).

Surgery

Since at least 90 percent of patients with back pain recover spontaneously in four to six weeks, surgery is usually not necessary. Most patients get better with minimal bed rest, an early return to normal activities, medications for relieving pain, and physical therapy or home exercises to strengthen the muscles supporting the back and abdomen. Using the 6 steps in the *Pain-Free Back Program*, along with the right medications, you should experience noticeable relief within days to a few weeks.

However, in some special circumstances surgery is considered. If your back pain is associated with incapacitating pain and disability, or loss of bladder or bowel control, further testing is needed. Or when an imaging test such as an X ray of the back, CT scan, or an MRI or myelogram (see page 171) shows an abnormality within the same area and type of pain you are describing, your doctor may refer you to a neurosurgeon or orthopedic surgeon. (Remember that an X ray, CT, or MRI may show abnormalities in up to 40 percent of people with no back pain at all!)

When to see a surgeon. The most common reason for seeing a surgeon is having aggravating pain that limits your activities, despite trying to manage the pain with the 6 steps in this program, medications, and time for healing. It may surprise you that finding a herniated disk, even with nerve compression, does not automatically mean you need surgery. Surgery is advised in only about 10 percent of cases. If you have worsening of numbness, tingling, or weakness in your legs or problems controlling your urine or bowels, then these are serious concerns and reasons to consider surgery. With an imaging test such as an X ray, CT, or MRI, your doctor can evaluate the results to see if the abnormality on the test matches the type of pain or neurological changes you describe to him or her. For example, if you have persistent lower back pain or sciatica even after six weeks of using the 6-step *Pain-Free Back Program*, you may benefit from an MRI to evaluate for an abnormality such as a ruptured disk.

Narrow the search. Your doctor will recommend either a neurosurgeon or orthopedic surgeon. A neurosurgeon specializes in surgery on the nervous system, including the brain and spinal cord; an orthopedic surgeon focuses on bone and joint surgery. Both perform surgery for ruptured disks. Once you have been given a referral, in this age of managed care, you must check to see if this surgeon will be accepted by your insurance provider.

Over the telephone, you can find out if the surgeon is board certified, which means the doctor passed a standard exam given by the governing board in his or her specialty. Your local medical society will tell you where the doctor went to medical school. (This should not necessarily be a determining factor, but if you've never heard of the school, you might want to do more research.) Sometimes it is a plus if the doctor is involved in any academic pursuits, such as teaching, writing, or research, as he may be more up to date in the latest developments in his field. It is important to know where the doctor has hospital privileges and where those hospitals are located. Some doctors may not admit patients to certain hospitals, and this is an important consideration, especially if you have chronic health problems. You should consider how many surgeries this physician has performed (25 to 30 would be minimum).

Plan a consultation. Once you have narrowed down your search, plan an initial consultation with the surgeon during which time you can get to know each other. This will include a detailed interview. Bring any previous test results with you, and talk openly about your needs. Ask what the chances are for pain relief. Be specific with questions about exercise and increasing activity. If you want to play golf or tennis, ask if it will be possible after disk removal surgery. If you cannot do your job that entails bending and lifting, ask if back surgery will help you at work. Patient-physician communication is important to receive the highest quality of care as well as comfort during the anxious moments prior to surgery.

Ask questions. Be sure to ask questions before the surgery, and have the surgeon describe what he or she is specifically planning to do. Before the surgery, you can be given a regional anesthesia, which numbs part of your body but allows you to remain awake. On the other hand, your surgeon may recommend general anesthesia, which puts you to sleep. Both types of anesthesia will prevent you from feeling pain.

Talk openly with your surgeon about the hospital stay, what you should expect as you recuperate from surgery, and the length of time it will take before you can be active again. Find assistance for day-to-day activities, particularly for the first few days after the procedure. Be sure to shower and wash your hair before the surgery, since it may be a while before you feel like doing this again. Some questions to consider asking your doctor include:

- Can you describe how the procedure will work?
- Can I be awake during the procedure?
- How much pain will I feel after surgery and for how long?
- How long will the rehabilitation last, and when can I be active again?
- What complications may occur and how can I avoid these?
- Are there certain measures that may help speed healing?

Talk about the intended outcome. Make sure you talk to your doctor about your expected goals from the back surgery. Discuss the risks of surgery, and be sure these are outweighed by the expected benefits. The goals usually involve relief of pain and more mobility and strength in the back and legs. If you have fears or concerns, now is the time to talk about these. You should feel comfortable and confident, because you trust these professionals.

Know what to expect after surgery. You may need to spend a couple of days in the hospital, although in some cases you might go home the same

Meet the Anesthesiologist

If your surgery is immediate, you may not have the chance to talk at length with your anesthesiologist. This professional maintains your life while the triggers for breathing are anesthetized. If you do not have the right amount of oxygen or if your blood pressure is not monitored, there could be a serious complication. If you are planning ahead for surgery, it is standard to meet with your anesthesiologist during the preoperative exam. Whether you meet a week ahead or five minutes before surgery, make sure the anesthesiologist knows the following:

- Health problems you may have (lung disease, heart problems, chronic illness)
- Previous problems with anesthesia in the past
- Your desire to be awake during surgery

Avoid Complications

You may sail through surgery like a breeze. Yet, even under the best of circumstances, certain complications might occur. This checklist can help you decide if a call to your doctor is warranted.
    Do you have ...

____   Muscle weakness
____   Muscle wasting
____   Decreased or loss of bladder function
____   Decreased or loss of bowel function
____   Urinary tract infection
____   Paralysis of the arm or leg
____   Wound infection
____   Decreased sexual function
____   Excessive bleeding
____   Signs of infection
____   Excessive pain
____   Fever

Any of these symptoms are *not normal* and would indicate that further treatment is warranted. Call your doctor immediately.

day as the procedure. Be sure to arrange a ride, since you might be drowsy from the anesthesia. After the surgery, you might feel some pain, numbness, or tingling with muscle spasm and inflammation. Make sure you are given a pain medication to help you get through the first days. Healing may take time, but with a positive attitude and the steps in the *Pain-Free Back Program*, you can easily speed your recovery. Be patient! If you are overweight, consider starting the Pain-Free Back weight-loss plan (see page 43) to return to a ideal body weight. This will decrease the load of work your back has to do to recover.

Use a Pain Calendar

A good test to help you determine if surgery is necessary is to chart the days when your back pain is immobilizing or keeps you from doing your daily tasks and activities. Use a calendar like the one below and every three weeks assess your pain. If more days are circled than not, or if the pain is not reduced, this may be an indication that surgery is warranted.

Pain Calendar						
1	2	3	4	5	6	7
8	9	10	11	12	13	14
15	16	17	18	19	20	21

Traditional Surgical Approaches for Back Pain

The following represent the most common surgical procedures for back pain:

Laminectomy. The most common surgery for the back is called a laminectomy. This is a type of back surgery used most often to treat a herniated disk. A herniated disk is a round cushion between the bones of your spine (vertebrae) that has bulged out from its proper place in your back. A herniated disk may press on nearby nerves and cause severe pain (sciatica).

With this procedure, the surgeon removes a small piece of bone from the back part of the vertebra, called the lamina. After the piece of bone is removed, the surgeon can then remove the ruptured part of the disk pressing on the nerves. This should decrease the pain caused by the herniated disk .

Nearly 80 to 90 percent of patients treated surgically will have good results. In 5 percent of patients, the pain will return. These patients may require another operation. Complications, including bleeding, nerve damage, or infection, are unusual if you select an experienced neurosurgeon. Unfortunately, some studies show that laminectomy itself can often lead to chronic low back pain.

Laminectomy is also used to treat lumbar stenosis, a narrowing of the spine that compresses nerves around it and causes a sciatic-type of pain (see page 178). With lumbar stenosis, you might have increasing pain in the back, which worsens during walking or leaning backwards (as in walking down a hill) and is relieved by leaning forward (stooping over or leaning on a grocery cart). Laminectomy is successful in relieving pain in about 80 to 90 percent of patients with lumbar stenosis. In most cases, surgery is the best option when pain medicines no longer work. After laminectomy for lumbar stenosis, most people resume their prior level of activity.

Fusion. Fusion is considered when there is instability of the spine because of severe inflammation and joint destruction of the cervical spine in the neck, as in rheumatoid arthritis. Fusing the bony vertebral bodies together will permanently restrict movement. Yet pain and overall function, as well as quality of life, can actually improve significantly. In some patients with different levels of laminectomy, fusion remains an option to reduce pain.

Fusion of the spine may relieve pain, when movement or position of the spine puts pressure on surrounding nerves, such as with spinal stenosis (narrowing of the spinal canal with age). Spondylolisthesis (slippage of

---

Self-Test for a Ruptured Disk

If you have back pain with pain down the leg, try the following self-test to see if a ruptured disk has possibly occurred: Lie flat on your bed, then raise your affected leg at the hip without bending your knee. Normally, you should be able to lift it straight up at a *90-degree* angle without pain. If you have pain in your back while doing this leg raise, you may have a ruptured disk. If there is numbness or tingling in the leg or foot, it could be a sign of nerve irritation. See your doctor for further advice.

one vertebral body on the one below it) can also be managed with fusion if the pain is incapacitating, which is rare.

With fusion of the spine, hardware (rods and screws) is placed to immobilize the spine, and often a piece of bone from another place in the body (a bone graft) is used to join the vertebrae together. Studies show that this procedure can help about 70 percent of those with this type of back pain.

Discectomy. This procedure involves surgery to remove a damaged disk. This can relieve pressure on the nerve. Discectomy has been done for several years, but the long-term results and benefits are not clear.

New surgical techniques are on the horizon to help safely resolve back pain. For example, using a laser or electricity to heat and shrink an injured disk is getting promising results in trials. Disk replacement, which entails removal of a damaged disk and replacing it with a disk prosthesis, is also under development. Implantations of electrodes, which electrically stimulate the spine, have received mixed results but are not routinely recommended at this time.

Treatment of Acute Vertebral Compression Fractures

Until recently, the only treatment for a compression fracture of the spine (discussed on page 176) was conservative therapy, including rest, pain medications, physical therapy, or back bracing. Although the pain may go away in a few weeks with this treatment, the chronic pain can be progressive, with muscle spasm around the deformity caused by the fracture. Also, with a compression fracture of the spine, the alignment of the spine changes and the actual loss of height can be dramatic, leading to what's called a dowager's hump. Over time, this leads to disabling pain, immobility, and increased number of hospital stays and even earlier death.

Two new procedures, considered minimally invasive, are found to treat severe back pain and disability with compression fractures from osteoporosis. (These are not meant for a vertebral compression fracture from a different cause, such as infection or cancer.)

Vertebroplasty. With this procedure, a long needle is put into the vertebra through the back, using guidance by CT or X ray to get to the correct spot in a collapsed vertebra. Bone cement (methylmethacrylate) is then injected into a vertebra for pain relief. This stabilizes the fracture and provides immediate pain relief in 90 to 100 percent of patients. By itself, however, vertebroplasty will not improve the deformity.

Kyphoplasty. Introduced in 1998, this procedure involves inflating a balloon inside the collapsed vertebra, before injecting the bone cement. The inflated balloon opens a cavity for the cement to fill and re-expands the compressed vertebra. This provides not only pain relief to 90 to 100 percent of patients but restores vertebral height in almost 70 percent of patients. (Reversing the loss of height is more successful in newer, more recent fractures.)

Studies show better pain relief immediately with kyphoplasty, even within the first 24 hours after the procedure. However, some evidence indicates no difference in pain in the long run between patients treated with vertebroplasty and those whose compression fractures are managed conservatively. This information is important, because we know most painful vertebral compression fractures will improve with conservative treatment in the first six weeks.

Of course, no surgical procedure is without possible complications. With these two surgeries, the long-term effects of cement in a vertebral body are not yet known. Complications occur in less than 10 percent of patients and include infection and nerve or spinal cord damage. Because the cement is injected under pressure, there is also a risk of leakage of bone cement into the spinal cord, muscle, or, rarely, into the bloodstream. The potential benefits of these two procedures are greater if pain persists for a couple of weeks after fracture, is not controlled with medications, or there is a noticeable loss of height. An obvious candidate for these procedures would be someone with several fractures causing a stooped posture, which could eventually be stooped so far over that it causes stomach pain or trouble breathing. If the timing of the fracture is unclear, and you are thinking about these two procedures, an MRI could help tell the age of the fracture.

It is also paramount to remember that though the new technology may appear impressive, the underlying osteoporosis itself must be treated—and another fracture of the spine or hip prevented. Once a fracture occurs, aggressive therapy is important for osteoporosis, as well as having a baseline test of bone mineral density. It's important to follow the 6 steps in your *Pain-Free Back Program*, particularly taking adequate calcium and vitamin D, avoiding risky activities, building muscle strength in the back and the supporting abdomen, and exercising regularly. In addition, a large percentage of people with osteoporosis are candidates for medications that improve the quality and amount of bone itself. Hip protectors can also lower the risk of hip fracture in a fall.

Managing Back Pain after Surgery

Immediately after an open surgery on the spine, a molded back brace is fitted to reduce any instability. If recommended, this brace will be pre-scribed by the surgeon. Otherwise, the goal is early return to low-impact activity as directed specifically by the surgeon and physical therapist. He or she will prescribe additional physical therapy and exercises that are crucial to resuming your daily activities as quickly as possible. Be sure to ask your doctor when you can return to specific activities, such as your exercise regimen or duties at work. If you are caring for children, make sure you have help available until your doctor allows you to safely lift again.

In addition to local healing of any surgical incision, the goal should include "preventive maintenance." The ideal way to approach recovery from a back surgery, in addition to adequate analgesia with medications prescribed by the surgeon or your physician, include:

1. *Treat the cause of the back pain.* For example, you have to treat the osteoporosis to prevent another fracture. Educating yourself on what osteoporosis is and then seeing your doctor for a bone mineral density (BMD) test if you are at risk are both important prevention measures. If your BMD is too low, make sure you get ample cal-cium and vitamin D, following the guidelines on page 176. Newer medications such as the bisphosphonates can actually increase BMD and decrease the chance of having another bone fracture. Contrary to what you might think, bed rest can actually lead to loss of bone mineral density, so slowly but gradually increase activity to prevent worsening osteoporosis.

2. *Decrease risk of falling.* You would hate to undergo successful back surgery, and then slip and fall at home while walking from the mail-box to the front door. Review the suggestions for fall-proofing your home (see page 114) and make sure your living environment won't add to your back pain.

3. *Continue the exercises in Step 1 that strengthen your back and trunk, including abdominal muscles that support your spine.* Low-impact exercises even after surgery, if directed by a physical therapist, may speed post-op recovery. Aquatics or water exercises are an ideal way to increase aerobic and strength after back surgery, with mini-mal force to the healing spine.

4. *Modify work activity.* Learn proper lifting techniques, as described on page 107. "Back school" may be an option, especially in a high-risk workplace, offered by experienced therapists. Corsets, or fitted back braces, do have a role in preventing back injury with repetitive lifting, twisting, or bending.

5. *Lose excess weight.* I know I've mentioned this several times, but this is most helpful before surgery to decrease surgical complications. It helps after surgery as well, to decrease the heavy load on the recovering back.

You must keep in mind after reading this chapter, that the outcome *without surgery* in at least 90 percent of patients with back pain is good. With or without surgery, you may get better on your own with time. After surgery is considered or even finished, education and *prevention* of another injury is paramount.

Comprehensive Pain Clinics

When Lucy's back surgery failed to correct the intractable spinal disk pain, she didn't know where else to turn. This forty-six-year-old woman had tried every pain medication, and though she got temporary relief from the five years of knee-buckling pain, it still came back and kept her from enjoying her life.

Lucy finally turned to a comprehensive pain clinic to seek help in managing her chronic back pain. Targeting the physical, emotional, intellectual, and social aspects of pain, health care professionals helped Lucy regain her quality of life and have hope once again.

If you've tried the 6-step *Pain-Free Back Program*, along with various medications and even surgery, yet still have unrelenting back pain, do not give up. A comprehensive pain clinic might help you to address the various symptoms and problems that pain causes in your life. For instance, you may have high levels of psychological distress, along with sleep disorders, inactivity, overeating, depression, and dissatisfaction with your relationships or work status—all because of back pain. Health-care professionals at a comprehensive pain clinic will give you suggestions for dealing with these issues appropriately. You will find that as each problem is isolated, and then discussed, accepted, and resolved, you may feel less pain and achieve a greater quality of life.

How to Choose a Pain Clinic

The American Chronic Pain Association recommends the following guidelines when evaluating a pain unit. For more information on choosing a multidisciplinary approach to pain management and to view a list of pain clinics across the United States, contact this organization at 800-533-3231 or go online at www.acpa.org.

1. Make sure you locate a legitimate program. Facilities that offer pain management should include several specific components, listed below.
   - The Commission on Accreditation of Rehabilitation Facilities (CARF) (800-444-8991) can provide you with a listing of accredited pain programs in your area (your health insurance may require that the unit be CARF accredited in order for you to receive reimbursement).
   - You can also contact the American Pain Society, a group of health care providers (708-966-5595), for additional information about pain units in your area.
2. Choose a good program that is convenient for you and your family. Many pain management programs do not offer outpatient care. Choosing a program close to your home will enable you to commute to the program each day.
3. Learn something about the people who run the program.
   - Try to meet several of the staff members to get a sense of the people you will be dealing with while on the unit.
   - The program should have a complete medical staff trained in pain management techniques, including:
     - Physician (may be a specialist from a different area but will have expertise in pain management)
     - Registered nurse
     - Psychiatrist or psychologist
     - Physical therapist
     - Occupational therapist
     - Biofeedback therapist
     - Family counselor
     - Vocational counselor
     - Personnel trained in pain management intervention

4. Make sure the program includes most of the following features:

Biofeedback training	Group therapy
Counseling	Occupational therapy
Family counseling	Assertiveness training
TENS units	Regional anesthesia (nerve blocks)

Physical therapy (exercise and body mechanics training, not massage, whirlpool, etc.)

Relaxation training and stress management

Educational program covering medications and other aspects of pain and its management

Aftercare (follow-up support once you have left the unit)

5. Be sure your family can be involved in your care.
   - Family members should be required to be involved in your treatment.
   - The program should provide special educational sessions for family members.
   - Joint counseling for you and your family should also be available.
6. Also, consider these additional factors:
   - What services will your insurance company reimburse, and what will you be expected to cover?
   - What is the unit's physical setup (is it in a patient care area or in an area by itself)?
   - What is the program's length of stay?
   - Is the program inpatient or outpatient (when going through medication detoxification, inpatient care is recommended)?
   - If you choose an out-of-town unit, can your family be involved in your care?
   - Do you understand what will be required of you during your stay (length of time you will be on unit, responsibility to take care of personal needs, etc.)?
   - Does the unit provide any type of job retraining?
   - Make sure that before they accept you the unit reviews your previous medical records and give you a complete physical evaluation to be sure you can participate in the program.

- Your personal physician can refer you to the unit, but many programs also accept self-referral.
- Obtain copies of your recent medical records to prevent duplicate testing.
- Try to talk with both present and past program participants to get their feedback about their stay on the unit.

There Are Answers!

Although the management of back pain remains a challenge to patients and doctors, I guarantee that this book will guide you in a pain-free direction. Using the many suggestions given in the *Pain-Free Back Program*, along with the myriad medications available and/or injections or surgical procedures, you can find the right treatment combination to get the most relief.

PART III

Pain-Free Back Recipes

Your Pain-Free Back Recipes are made with the same healing foods and nutrients discussed in Step 2. For instance, antioxidants and phytochemicals found in fresh vegetables and fruits are important to keep your immune system working efficiently. Soy products keep bones strong and might even help you feel less pain, according to a new study discussed on page 57. Omega-3 fatty acids found in salmon, tuna fish, and olive oil help to reduce inflammation—and as you know, many times back pain stems from inflammation. Enzymes found in pineapple also help to decrease inflammatory action—and I cannot think of a more delicious fruit than pineapple!

Whether you are a meat eater, vegetarian, or someone who wants to cut back on carbs to drop a few pounds, these recipes will help you to reduce inflammation, keep bones strong, and even lose weight, if you carefully follow the instructions on page 43. All of the recipes are relatively low in saturated fat and calories, and we have put an asterisk (*) next to those recipes that are also low in carbohydrates.

Categories

Drinks and Appetizers
Tropical Smoothie
Twelve-Layer Bean Dip*

Salads and Sauces
Pesto Sauce*
Peanut Sauce*
Mandarin Orange Salad with
    Almonds*
Tropical Fruit Salad
Lin's Potato Salad with Vibrant
    Veggies*
Spinach Salad with Prosciutto*

Soups
Gram's Veggie Chili
Indian Lentil Dal
Gazpacho*
Curry Butternut Squash Soup

Breads
Peanut Butter Banana
    Muffins*
Almond Pancakes with
    Strawberries
Italian Garlic Bread
Almond Pumpkin Loaf

Pasta and Rice
Angel Hair with Shrimp, Goat
    Cheese, and Tomatoes
Authentic Pesto Pasta with
    Broccoli
Egg and Vegetable Fried Rice
Thai Noodles with Tofu and
    Veggies
Penne with Sun-Dried Tomato
    Pesto
Claire's Paella

Entrees
Asian Chicken Salad*
Chicken Pot Pie
Open-Faced Tuna Sandwiches*
Pecan-Crusted Salmon Bites*
Salmon with Dill Sauce*

---

*Low in carbohydrates.

Entrees *(continued)*
Zesty Meat Loaf*
Sloppy Joe Mixture*
Retro Macaroni and Cheese
Black-Eyed Peas and Greens*
Creamed Chicken with Tortillas*
Mediterranean Soft Tacos*
Grilled Portobello Sandwiches
   with Goat Cheese

Sautéed Kale with Feta*
Dharma's Collard Greens*
Baked Peas with Cheese*
Lemon-Ginger Carrots*
Roasted Sweet Potatoes and
   Winter Squash with Rosemary
Healthy Fries
Barbecued Tofu*
Soy Sausage Balls*

Vegetables/Sides
Guacamole*
Summer Salsa*
Tasty Green Beans*
Rapini with Garlic and Pine Nuts*

Desserts
Pineapple Upside-Down Cake
Healthy Carrot Cake
Tasty Tofu Cake
Nut Meringue Cookies*

DRINKS AND APPETIZERS

❖ Tropical Smoothie

Ingredients
1 cup fresh pineapple, diced
2 medium bananas, diced
1 cup frozen mango, diced
2 tablespoons flaxseed, ground
2 cups low-fat milk

Directions
Place all ingredients in a blender. Mix until fruit is completely blended. Serve immediately.

Yield: Serves 2.

Nutrition information per serving: Calories: 374; Fat: 8g; Carbohydrates: 69g; Fiber: 9g; Protein: 14g.

---

*Low in carbohydrates.

✤ Twelve-Layer Bean Dip*

Ingredients
1 15-ounce can refried beans
1 15-ounce can black beans, rinsed and drained
1 cup guacamole (see page 247)
1 cup low-fat sour cream
2 cups shredded lettuce
1 cup shredded cheddar cheese
1 cup Summer Salsa (see page 247)
¼ cup black olives, chopped
¼ cup cilantro, chopped
½ cup Roma tomatoes, chopped
1 green onion, sliced
Jalapeno peppers, optional

Directions
Prepare guacamole and Summer Salsa according to recipes in this section. You can also substitute store-bought guacamole and salsa. In a large, deep serving dish, spread refried beans. Sprinkle black beans over the refried beans. On top of this, spread the guacamole. Spread sour cream on top, and then add lettuce, cheese, and olives. Top with salsa, cilantro, tomatoes, and green onion. Season to taste and add jalapeno peppers, if desired. Serve with tortilla chips or raw veggie sticks.

Yield: Serves 6.

Nutrition information per serving: Calories: 170; Fat: 6g; Carbohydrates: 26g; Fiber: 8g; Protein: 10g.

SALADS AND SAUCES

✣ Pesto Sauce*

Ingredients
2 large garlic cloves
2 cups packed fresh basil leaves
3 tablespoons pine nuts
4 tablespoons fresh Parmesan cheese
⅓ cup olive oil

Directions
Blend ingredients in a food processor. Add more olive oil to taste for a smoother consistency.

Yield: Serves 4.

Nutrition information per serving: Calories: 224; Fat: 2g; Carbohydrates: 3g; Fiber: 2g; Protein: 4g.

✣ Peanut Sauce*

Ingredients
1 tablespoon canola oil
1 clove garlic, minced
¼ cup onion, finely chopped
3 tablespoons peanut butter
¼ cup water
1 teaspoon rice vinegar
1 tablespoon soy sauce
1 teaspoon honey
1 teaspoon fresh ginger, minced
½ teaspoon garlic powder
½ teaspoon onion powder
¼ teaspoon cayenne pepper

Directions
Heat oil in a small saucepan. Sauté onion and garlic on medium heat for 3–4 minutes until translucent. Add peanut butter and stir until melted.

Add the rest of the ingredients and stir. Simmer for several minutes until thick and creamy. For a smoother sauce, blend mixture in a food processor. You may wish to add more water for a thinner sauce.

Yield: Serves 2.

Nutrition information per serving: Calories: 224; Fat: 20g; Carbohydrates: 9g; Fiber: 1g; Protein: 7g.

❖ Mandarin Orange Salad with Almonds*

Ingredients
1 head of premium Boston lettuce
   (about 4 cups)
1 large carrot, finely grated
1 cup mandarin orange slices, halved
¼ cup almonds, slivered

DRESSING
4 tablespoons orange juice
4 tablespoons vegetable oil
3 tablespoons rice vinegar
1 tablespoon honey
Salt, to taste

Directions
Tear lettuce into bite-sized pieces. Toss lettuce with carrots, mandarin oranges, and almonds. Combine dressing ingredients in a separate bowl. Whisk lightly. Toss salad with dressing just before serving.

Yield: Serves 4.

Nutrition information per serving: Calories: 192; Fat: 17g; Carbohydrates: 10g; Fiber: 2g; Protein: 3g.

❖ Tropical Fruit Salad

Ingredients
1 pineapple, cored, diced in small squares
2 mangoes, peeled, cored, diced
1 papaya, peeled, seeded, diced
2 navel oranges, peeled, diced
4 kiwis, peeled, sliced
¼ cup orange juice
¼ cup shredded, unsweetened coconut
½ cup golden raisins

Directions
Prepare fruit and combine in large serving bowl. Before serving, pour orange juice over salad and toss well. Add coconut and raisins.

Yield: Serves 6.

Nutrition information per serving: Calories: 247; Fat: 7g; Carbohydrates: 50g; Fiber: 8g; Protein: 3g.

❖ Lin's Potato Salad with Vibrant Veggies*

Ingredients
2 cups prepared potato salad
1 head red leaf lettuce, washed
1 fresh tomato, diced
1 avocado, diced
1 stalk celery, diced
1 medium carrot, grated
½ red onion, finely chopped
1 red pepper, diced
1 cucumber, peeled, sliced
½ cup green and/or black olives
½ cup chickpeas
½ cup canned corn, drained
1 cup feta cheese, crumbled

RED WINE VINAIGRETTE DRESSING

½ cup canola oil
¼ cup red wine vinegar
2 tablespoons Parmesan cheese
½ tablespoon sugar
½ teaspoon salt
½ teaspoon celery salt
¼ teaspoon pepper
½ teaspoon dry mustard
1 garlic clove, minced
¼ teaspoon paprika

Directions

Spread whole red lettuce leaves on a large platter. Spoon potato salad in center of platter on top of leaves. Artfully, spread the remaining salad ingredients around the potato salad. Combine all dressing ingredients and mix well. Pour dressing over the salad and vegetables and serve immediately.

Yield: Serves 7.

Nutrition information per serving: Calories: 431; Fat: 28g; Carbohydrates: 26g; Fiber: 6g; Protein: 6g.

❖ Spinach Salad with Prosciutto*

Ingredients

6 cups fresh spinach, washed,
    drained in paper towels
2 cups fresh basil leaves, washed,
    drained in paper towels
⅓ cup olive oil
3 cloves garlic, finely chopped
½ cup pine nuts
¾ cup prosciutto, chopped finely
¾ cup Parmesan cheese

Directions

Spread pine nuts in a single layer on a pan. Cook at 250 degrees for 5–10 minutes, watching carefully for browning. Make sure they do not burn. Place garlic and oil in a pan on medium heat, then add prosciutto. Sauté several minutes, until cooked through. Remove from heat and cool for five minutes. Add prosciutto mixture to spinach and basil, and toss gently. Add Parmesan and serve immediately.

Yield: Serves 4.

Nutrition information per serving: Calories: 383; Fat: 32g; Carbohydrates: 7g; Fiber: 3g; Protein: 19g.

SOUPS

✢ Gram's Veggie Chili

Ingredients

3 tablespoons canola oil
1 large onion, chopped
1 large green pepper, chopped
1 clove garlic, minced
1 package soy crumbles (or substitute 1 pound
    green beef, if preferred)
2 15-ounce cans chili beans with seasonings
1 15-ounce can tomato sauce
2 cups hot water
1 cup carrots, finely chopped
1 tablespoon sugar

Directions

In a small sauté pan, sauté onion, green pepper, and garlic in 1 tablespoon of oil on medium heat until soft. In a large saucepan, sauté soy burger crumbles in 2 tablespoons oil on medium heat until cooked through, about 5–10 minutes. Add beans, tomato sauce, water, carrots, and sugar. Bring to a boil. Simmer for 30 minutes. Add more water if chili is too thick. Serve with sour cream, green onions, or shredded cheese. Top with jalapenos.

Yield: Serves 4.

Nutrition information per serving: Calories: 400; Fat: 13g; Carbohydrates: 67g; Fiber: 13g; Protein: 23g.

❖ Indian Lentil Dal

Ingredients
2 tablespoons oil
1 cup uncooked red lentils, rinsed
1 onion, finely chopped
½ tablespoon fresh ginger
1 jalapeno, minced
¼ tablespoon cumin
¼ tablespoon garam masala
½ teaspoon turmeric
½ teaspoon cayenne pepper
½ teaspoon sugar
½ teaspoon salt

Directions
Place oil in large saucepan on medium high. Add lentils, onions, ginger, and jalapeno. Stir and let cook for one minute. Add water to pot. Cover and let simmer for 1–2 hours on medium heat. Add seasonings. Dal is ready when lentils are very soft and creamy. Serve with rice and a dollop of plain yogurt.

Yield: Serves 4.

Nutrition information per serving: Calories: 236; Fat: 8g; Carbohydrates: 31g; Fiber: 6g; Protein: 12g.

✤ Gazpacho*

Ingredients
1 small onion
2 medium cucumbers, peeled
1 medium green bell pepper
5 large tomatoes, peeled and seeded
16 ounces tomato juice
1 large tomato (for tomato stock)
5 cloves garlic
⅓ cup olive oil
¾ teaspoon chili powder
½ cup fresh cilantro, chopped, for garnish
Jalapeno pepper, optional

Directions
Chop all vegetables (except the tomato for the stock) into very small squares. (Vegetables should be cut in uniform pieces for best presentation.) Place cut vegetables in a large bowl. Add 4 ounces tomato juice, the tomato for the stock, garlic, chili powder, and olive oil to blender and mix until smooth. Pour over vegetables in the bowl. Stir. Add remaining tomato juice in increments of 2 ounces until desired consistency is reached. Chill at least two hours before serving, or overnight. Add salt and pepper to taste just before serving. Garnish with cilantro and jalapeno.

Yield: Serves 4.

Nutrition information per serving: Calories: 247; Fat: 17g; Carbohydrates: 18g; Fiber: 4g; Protein: 3g.

❖ Curry Butternut Squash Soup

Ingredients
2 medium butternut squash (about 3 cups)
1 large baking potato
1 tablespoon canola oil
1 large onion, diced
2 cups water
¼ teaspoon fresh ground nutmeg
¼ teaspoon oregano
½ teaspoon garlic powder
1 teaspoon curry powder
1 cup apple juice
1 cup low-fat milk

Directions
Bake squash and potato at 350 degrees for 30 minutes. Let cool for 30 minutes, and then peel the vegetables. Scoop the flesh from the butternut squash and discard the seeds and strings. Sauté onion in oil in a large saucepan on medium heat. Cook several minutes, and then add squash and potato. Cook for several more minutes. Add water and seasonings and bring to a boil. Cover pot and simmer, stirring occasionally, for 10 minutes. Add mixture to blender and pulse until creamy. Add apple juice and milk, and simmer an additional 5–10 minutes. Add salt and pepper to taste and garnish with green onions, chopped walnuts, or sour cream.

Yield: Serves 4.

Nutrition information per serving: Calories: 221; Fat: 4g; Carbohydrates: 42g; Fiber: 4g; Protein: 6g.

BREADS

❖ Peanut Butter Banana Muffins*

Ingredients
2 tablespoons protein powder
    (optional)
1 cup all-purpose flour
¾ cup Quaker oats
⅓ cup brown sugar
1 tablespoon baking powder
1 cup low-fat milk
2 cups ripe banana, mashed
1 egg, beaten
3 tablespoons canola oil
2 cups peanut butter
1 teaspoon vanilla

Directions
Preheat oven to 375 degrees. Grease two 12-muffin pans with oil or line
with paper baking cups. Combine protein powder, flour, oats, brown
sugar, and baking powder in a large bowl. In a separate bowl, whisk
together milk, banana, egg, oil, peanut butter, and vanilla. Add to dry
ingredients, mixing until just blended. Refrigerate at least two hours. Fill
prepared muffin cups three-quarters full. Bake 16 minutes or until
cooked through.

Yield: 24 muffins.

Nutrition information per serving: Calories: 210; Fat: 14g; Carbohydrates:
17g; Fiber: 2g; Protein: 9g.

❖ Almond Pancakes with Strawberries

Ingredients
¾ cup all-purpose flour
¼ cup whole-wheat flour
1 tablespoon sugar
2 teaspoons baking powder
1 teaspoon salt
1 large egg, beaten
1 cup low-fat milk
3 tablespoons ground almonds
1 cup fresh strawberries, sliced
Canola oil for cooking pancakes

Directions
Heat oil in a large pan or on a griddle. Combine all ingredients except strawberries. Stir just until blended. Pour batter onto oiled pan. Cook until bottoms of pancakes are golden brown, then flip. Serve with fresh strawberries on top.

Yield: Serves 3.

Nutrition information per serving: Calories: 286; Fat: 7g; Carbohydrates: 45g; Fiber: 4g; Protein: 12g.

❖ Italian Garlic Bread

Ingredients
1 small loaf Italian bread (about 8 slices)
¾ cup Parmesan cheese
½ teaspoon salt
½ teaspoon pepper
½ teaspoon dried basil
1 teaspoon dried oregano
1 teaspoon dried chives
2 large garlic cloves, chopped finely
4 tablespoons olive oil

Directions

Combine all seasonings with olive oil and Parmesan cheese. Mix well. Slice loaf into 8 slices. Spoon garlic mixture onto slices of bread, spreading evenly. Re-form loaf and wrap in aluminum foil. Bake at 350 degrees for 10–15 minutes. Bake longer for crispier bread.

Yield: Serves 4.

Nutrition information per serving: Calories: 370; Fat: 16g; Carbohydrates: 32g; Fiber: 2g; Protein: 13g.

✤ Almond Pumpkin Loaf

Ingredients

3¼ cups flour
2 teaspoons baking soda
1¼ teaspoon salt
1 teaspoon ground cinnamon
½ teaspoon fresh ground nutmeg
½ teaspoon ground cloves
2 cups pumpkin (canned or fresh)
4 eggs
¾ cup vegetable oil
½ cup applesauce
½ cup water
2 cups white sugar
1 cup brown sugar
½ cup ground almonds

Directions

Preheat oven to 350. Grease three loaf pans (each about 7 x 3 inches each). Sift flour, baking soda, salt, cinnamon, nutmeg, and cloves until well combined. In a separate bowl, blend pumpkin, eggs, oil, applesauce, water, sugar, and ground almonds. Add dry ingredients to batter. Mix well. Pour batter into loaf pans and bake 50–60 minutes. Breads will be finished when inserted toothpick comes out clean.

Yield: 24 slices.

Nutrition information per serving: Calories: 238; Fat: 9g; Carbohydrates: 41g; Fiber: 2g; Protein: 3g.

PASTA AND RICE

❖ Angel Hair with Shrimp, Goat Cheese and Tomatoes

Ingredients
8 ounces whole-wheat angel hair pasta
2 tablespoons olive oil
1 pound fresh shrimp, shelled and deveined
4 cloves garlic, peeled and minced
1 tablespoon fresh lemon juice
6 ounces goat cheese, crumbled
4 small Roma tomatoes, diced in small squares
1 tablespoon fresh parsley

Directions
Cook pasta according to package directions, then drain. Heat olive oil in a large skillet on medium-high. Add shrimp and cook 4–5 minutes, or until shrimp turn opaque. Sprinkle with lemon juice and throw in the garlic. Cook an additional minute or two, on medium-low, until garlic turns golden. Remove from heat. Toss pasta, shrimp, and Roma tomatoes. Add salt to taste. Top with goat cheese and parsley.

Yield: Serves 4.

Nutrition information per serving: Calories: 433; Fat: 17g; Carbohydrates: 48g; Fiber: 6g; Protein: 17g.

❖ Authentic Pesto Pasta with Broccoli

Ingredients
Authentic Pesto, see page 220
8 ounces whole-wheat thin spaghetti
2 cups fresh broccoli, washed, cut into bite-sized pieces

Directions
Prepare pesto according to recipe. Boil pasta and cook according to pack-age directions. While pasta is cooking, heat ¼ cup water in a saucepan. Heat to boil, and then add broccoli and cover. Steam broccoli on medium heat for 3–4 minutes until crisp-tender. Drain broccoli. When spaghetti is done, drain in a colander. In a large bowl, toss pasta, broccoli, and pesto until well combined. Add salt and pepper to taste. Top with Parmesan cheese and serve with garlic bread.

Yield: Serves 4.

Nutrition information per serving: Calories: 269; Fat: 5g; Carbohydrates: 46g; Fiber: 7g; Protein: 5g.

❖ Egg and Vegetable Fried Rice

Ingredients
2½ cups quick-cooking rice
2 tablespoons canola oil
1 large onion, peeled and chopped
1 carrot, finely chopped
1 green pepper, finely chopped
2 scallions, finely chopped
1 teaspoon ginger, minced
2 cloves garlic, minced
1 9-ounce package frozen green peas
3 eggs
1 teaspoon sugar
3 tablespoons soy sauce

Directions
Heat 4 cups of water to boiling. Add ½ teaspoon salt and the rice. Cook for 10 minutes, until tender. Drain rice completely and spread on a large platter to dry. Heat 2 tablespoons oil and add onion, carrot, green pepper, scallions, and ginger. Stir-fry for 4–5 minutes until onion is translucent and carrot begins to soften. Beat the eggs. Pour the egg into the pan, pouring in a thin stream. Stir veggies while adding the eggs, so that the egg breaks into small pieces. Cook another 2–3 minutes, until egg hardens. Add rice, sugar, and soy sauce. Continue cooking, stirring occasionally. If rice is sticking to the pan, add more oil.

Yield: Serves 5.

Nutrition information per serving: Calories: 289; Fat: 10g; Carbohydrates: 41g; Fiber: 6g; Protein: 10g.

❖ Thai Noodles with Tofu and Veggies

Ingredients
3 tablespoons canola oil
1 block of extra firm tofu
   (16 ounces)
1 tablespoon honey
1 tablespoon soy sauce
½ tablespoon garlic powder
1 small onion
1 cup snow peas or sugar
   snap peas, washed
1 small red pepper, washed and diced
2 cloves garlic, minced
1 teaspoon fresh ginger, minced
8 ounces rice noodles
Peanut Sauce, double recipe,
   see page 220

Directions

In a large sauté pan, heat 2 tablespoons of the oil on medium-high heat. Chop tofu into small rectangles, about 1 inch wide by 2 inches long and ½ inch thick. Add tofu to pan and fry for 3–4 minutes, and then flip after the first side is golden brown. Fry second side of tofu, drizzling honey and soy sauce directly over the tofu. Cook for 3-4 minutes until both sides of tofu are golden brown. Remove from heat and drain on paper towels. Sprinkle with garlic powder.

Cook rice noodles according to package directions, then drain. Add remaining 1 tablespoon of oil to a sauté pan. Add chopped onion. While onion is cooking, trim ends of snow or sugar snap peas. When onion is translucent, add peas, red pepper, ginger and garlic. Sauté for 3 minutes. Prepare peanut sauce. Once vegetables are crisp-tender, add peanut sauce and noodles to vegetables. Toss to combine.

Yield: Serves 5.

Nutrition information per serving: Calories: 448; Fat: 22g; Carbohydrates: 50g; Fiber: 5g; Protein: 16g.

❖ Penne with Sun-Dried Tomato Pesto

Ingredients
8 ounces penne pasta
2 tablespoons tomato paste
⅓ cup sun-dried tomatoes
2 cloves garlic
¼ cup fresh mint leaves, washed
⅓ cup walnuts
¼ cup olive oil
2 tablespoons water, or more,
    as needed
4 ounces feta cheese, crumbled

Directions
Cook pasta according to package directions, then drain. Set aside to cool. Reconstitute sun-dried tomatoes by heating ½ cup of water in a pot. Bring to a boil. Add tomatoes to the water and turn off the heat. Allow toma-

toes to soak for at least 5 minutes, then drain on paper towels. Place sun-dried tomatoes, garlic, mint, walnuts, and olive oil in a food processor and blend until well mixed. You may need to add water, a teaspoon at a time, for better consistency. Once mixed, toss penne with sun-dried tomato pesto. Top with feta cheese.

Yield: Serves 4.

Nutrition information per serving: Calories: 467; Fat: 26g; Carbohydrates: 49g; Fiber: 8g; Protein: 19g.

❖ Claire's Paella

Ingredients
2 tablespoons olive oil
1 pound chicken breasts, boneless, skinless, cut into bite-sized pieces
8 ounces pork, cut into bite-sized pieces
1 small onion, diced
1 green pepper, diced
3 cloves garlic, minced
1 cup green beans, washed, diced
    into 1-inch pieces
1 large tomato, seeded and diced
3½ cups chicken or vegetable broth
2 cups Spanish or yellow rice (uncooked)
¼ teaspoon dried saffron, crushed
½ teaspoon turmeric
Juice of one lemon
Salt and pepper to taste

Directions
Heat olive oil in a large skillet on medium heat. Add chicken and pork and cook until they begin to brown, about 10–15 minutes. Add onion and sauté for two minutes. Add green pepper, garlic, and green beans and continue to cook for several minutes. Add tomato and stir well, cooking until liquid is mostly absorbed. Turn heat up to high and add broth to skillet. Bring to a boil and stir in rice. When broth is boiling, add saffron and turmeric. Boil for 5 minutes. Do not stir after this point. Lower heat and

simmer for 15–20 minutes or until rice is cooked and liquid is fully absorbed. Drizzle lemon juice over paella before serving.

Yield: Serves 5.

Nutrition information per serving: Calories: 450; Fat: 3g; Carbohydrates: 68g; Fiber: 4g; Protein: 23g.

ENTREES

✤ Asian Chicken Salad*

Ingredients
1 tablespoon canola or sesame oil
2 boneless, skinless chicken breasts
2 cloves garlic, minced
1 tablespoon fresh ginger, minced
2 green onions, diced
1 stalk celery, diced
1 carrot, steamed, diced
2 tablespoons rice wine vinegar or white vinegar
¼ cup chicken broth
2 tablespoons soy sauce
Dash of crushed red pepper

DRESSING
2 tablespoons light mayonnaise
1 tablespoon rice wine vinegar
1 tablespoon canola or sesame oil
1 teaspoon garlic powder
½ teaspoon dried lemongrass

Directions
Place chicken breasts in pan with 1 tablespoon canola oil. Cook on medium-high heat for several minutes. Flip, then cover and steam for 6–7

minutes or until cooked through. Set aside to cool. Place garlic, ginger, green onions, celery, and carrot in sauté pan on medium-high heat. Add vinegar, chicken broth, soy sauce, and a crushed red pepper to taste. Cook for several minutes until liquid is mostly absorbed. Combine dressing ingredients in a large bowl and mix well. Cut chicken into small bite-sized pieces and add to dressing. Toss in vegetable mixture and mix well. Serve warm or cold.

Yield: Serves 5.

Nutrition information per serving: Calories: 188; Fat: 9g; Carbohydrates: 3g; Fiber: <1g; Protein: 22g.

❖ Chicken Pot Pie

FILLING
1 tablespoon butter
1 tablespoon canola oil
1 cup cooked, boneless, skinless
    chicken breasts, diced
1 medium carrot, steamed,
    cut into tiny triangles
¼ cup onion, diced
10 ounces frozen peas
1 cup cooked potatoes,
    chopped into small squares

SAUCE
4 tablespoons unsalted butter
4 tablespoons all-purpose flour
1½ cups chicken or vegetable stock
⅓ cup half-and-half
½ teaspoon salt
½ teaspoon pepper

CRUST
2 frozen piecrusts
1 egg white

Directions

Heat a large skillet over medium heat and add 1 tablespoon butter and 1 tablespoon canola oil. Sauté onions for several minutes until translucent. Add carrots, potatoes, and peas. Cook until warm and vegetables are soft. Place vegetables in large bowl and set aside. In the same pan, melt 3 tablespoons of butter. Whisk in flour and stir for several minutes as the sauce thickens. Once smooth, remove sauce from heat and whisk in half-and-half, milk, salt and pepper. Return mixture to heat. Continue stirring, and simmer. Once the mixture is creamy and thick, add chicken and vegetables. Set the filling aside and cool while preparing pie crusts.

Allow piecrusts to thaw for several minutes. Take one pie shell and cut off the crimped edge with a sharp knife. This will be the top crust of the pie. Take the other crust, still in the metal pie pan, and add the cooled filling. Then place the top crust over the pie and gently remove metal pie pan. With fingers, press edges of the pie shells together until edges are completely sealed. Make several slits in the top crust with a knife. Brush the top of the crust with the egg white. Bake chicken pot pie according to the directions on the packaging.

Yield: Serves 6.

Nutrition information per serving: Calories: 444; Fat: 28g; Carbohydrates: 35g; Fiber: 4g; Protein: 18g.

✣ Open-Faced Tuna Sandwiches

Ingredients

12 ounces canned, water-packed,
　　white tuna, drained
3 tablespoons light mayonnaise
1 tablespoon light cream cheese
1 stalk celery, diced in small squares
¼ cup red onion, diced in small squares
Juice of one lemon
2 tablespoons sweet gherkins, finely chopped
8 slices whole wheat bread
6 ounces cheddar cheese, grated or sliced
Salt and pepper to taste

Directions
Combine tuna, mayonnaise, cream cheese, celery, and red onion. Mix well. Add lemon juice and gherkins, stir. Add salt and fresh ground pepper. Lightly toast bread until golden. Spoon tuna salad on top of toast and top with cheese. Put in oven and bake at 375 degrees until cheese is melted. Serve warm.

Yield: Serves 4.

Nutrition information per serving: Calories: 495; Fat: 22g; Carbohydrates: 33g; Fiber: 5g; Protein: 38g.

❖ Pecan-Crusted Salmon Bites*

Ingredients
1 pound salmon filets
½ cup pecans, finely chopped
1 teaspoon sugar
Salt to taste
2 tablespoons orange juice
1 egg white

Directions
Remove bones from salmon and cut into small squares. Place salmon on a greased baking sheet with sides touching. Bake salmon at 425 degrees for 10 minutes. Combine pecans, sugar, salt, orange juice, and egg white. Take salmon out of oven and pour pecan topping evenly over salmon. Bake for an additional 10 minutes or until cooked through.

Yield: Serves 4.

Nutrition information per serving: Calories: 289; Fat: 19g; Carbohydrates: 5g; Fiber: 1g; Protein: 27g.

❖ Salmon with Dill Sauce*

Ingredients
2 tablespoons olive oil
1 tablespoon white wine or white vinegar
Juice of 2 lemons
¼ cup green onions, chopped
2 cloves garlic, minced
Pinch of red pepper
⅔ cup low-fat sour cream
4 tablespoons fresh dill, chopped
1 pound salmon filets

Directions
Combine olive oil, vinegar, lemon juice, green onions, garlic, and red pepper. Add salt and pepper to taste. Place salmon in baking dish and pour marinade over fish. Cover with plastic wrap and refrigerate salmon for at least three hours. Flip salmon filets and spoon marinade over fish several times. After several hours, place individual filets in pieces of aluminum foil. Cover each piece with the marinade and wrap foil around filets. Cook for 20–30 minutes at 350 degrees until cooked through. Mix sour cream and dill. After baking, spoon sour cream mixture over fish. Serve immediately.

Yield: Serves 4.

Nutrition information per serving: Calories: 300; Fat: 20g; Carbohydrates: 4g; Fiber: <1g; Protein: 26g.

❖ Zesty Meat Loaf*

Ingredients
1 pound ground beef
¾ cup whole-wheat bread crumbs
½ cup onion, finely chopped
1 egg
2 teaspoons garlic powder
1 teaspoon Worcestershire sauce
¼ cup plain tomato sauce
2 tablespoons tomato paste
2 tablespoons brown sugar
2 tablespoons pineapple preserves
¼ cup pineapple, crushed
Salt and pepper to taste

Directions
Preheat oven to 350 degrees. Mix ground beef, bread crumbs, onion, egg, garlic powder and Worcestershire sauce. Stir until well blended. Add salt and pepper to taste. Place in loaf pan and bake for 45 minutes. While the loaf is baking, pulse tomato sauce, tomato paste, sugar, and pineapple ingredients in a food processor just until blended. After loaf cooks for 45 minutes, pour tomato glaze over it. Return to oven and cook for an additional 10–20 minutes or until cooked through.

Yield: Serves 4.

Nutrition information per serving: Calories: 282; Fat: 8g; Carbohydrates: 26g; Fiber: 2g; Protein: 26g.

✤ Sloppy Joe Mixture*

Ingredients
2 tablespoons olive oil
1 pound ground beef
1 onion, diced
2 medium green peppers, diced
1 16-ounce can tomato sauce
1 tablespoon chili powder
1 teaspoon garlic powder
1 teaspoon dried mustard
½ teaspoon oregano
2 tablespoons brown sugar

Directions
Heat ground beef in 1 tablespoon oil on medium heat. Cook, stirring occasionally, until browned. Heat onion and green pepper in 1 tablespoon oil and stir, cooking on medium heat for several minutes. Add beef, vegetables, tomato sauce, and seasonings to large sauce pan. Simmer for 15 minutes, stirring, until well combined. Serve on whole-wheat hamburger buns.

Yield: Serves 4.

Nutrition information per serving: Calories: 296; Fat: 13g; Carbohydrates: 21g; Fiber: 3g; Protein: 25g.

❖ Retro Macaroni and Cheese

Ingredients
½ pound elbow macaroni
2 tablespoons butter
2 tablespoons flour
1½ tablespoons powdered mustard
2 cups low-fat milk
¾ cup half-and-half
1 large egg
10 ounces sharp cheddar cheese, shredded
½ cup low-fat ricotta cheese
1 teaspoon salt
Fresh black pepper, ground, to taste

TOPPING
3 tablespoons butter
1 cup bread crumbs

Directions
Preheat oven to 350. Cook pasta according to package directions. In large saucepan, add butter and melt over medium heat. Add flour and whisk until butter is smooth, stirring for several minutes. Add 8 ounces of cheddar and all of the ricotta cheese. Slowly stir in the egg. Allow to simmer 2 more minutes, until well blended. Pour mixture into large baking dish. Top with 2 ounces of cheese, salt and pepper. For the topping, melt 3 tablespoons butter and mix with bread crumbs. Gently spread on top of macaroni. Bake, uncovered, for 30 minutes until liquid is absorbed and topping is crispy.

Yield: Serves 7.

Nutrition information per serving: Calories: 440; Fat: 28g; Carbohydrates: 37g; Fiber: 2g; Protein: 22g.

❖ Black-Eyed Peas and Greens*

Ingredients
1 tablespoon olive oil
1 onion, chopped
8 cups of raw collard greens
1 clove garlic, finely chopped
2 tablespoons red wine vinegar
2 tablespoons water
2 15-ounce cans black-eyed peas, rinsed, drained
Hot sauce, optional
Salt and pepper to taste

Directions
Place olive oil and onion in a large pan on medium heat. Sauté onion until translucent. Add collard greens, garlic, and vinegar to pan, stirring constantly. Cook, adding water if necessary. Once greens start to wilt, add black-eyed peas and seasonings. Cook on medium heat until cooked through.

Yield: Serves 6.

Nutrition information per serving: Calories: 163; Fat: 4g; Carbohydrates: 26g; Fiber: 10g; Protein: 4g.

❖ Creamed Chicken with Tortillas*

Ingredients
6 6-inch whole wheat tortillas
3 cups chicken, cooked, chopped
1 can low-fat cream of mushroom soup
¼ cup cilantro, chopped
4 ounces light cream cheese
½ cup onion, chopped
1 cup spinach, chopped
½ teaspoon cumin
1 teaspoon garlic powder
1 tomato, diced
8 ounces Monterey jack or cheddar cheese
Salt and pepper to taste

Directions

Heat oven to 350 degrees. Cut tortillas into long strips about 1 inch wide. Set aside. Combine chicken, soup, cilantro, cream cheese, onion, spinach, cumin, and garlic powder. Mix well. Pour half of the chicken mixture into the baking pan. Cover with half of the tortilla strips. Pour the rest of the chicken mixture over the tortilla strips. Top with tortilla strips. Spread cheese and tomatoes over the top of the dish. Bake, covered, for 30 minutes. Remove foil and then bake for an additional 10–15 minutes until fully cooked.

Yield: Serves 6.

Nutrition information per serving: Calories: 444; Fat: 23g; Carbohydrates: 24g; Fiber: 3g; Protein: 34g.

❖ Mediterranean Soft Tacos*

Ingredients

1 teaspoon olive oil
1 small onion, chopped
2 fresh garlic cloves, minced
10 ounces spinach, torn into small pieces
4 ounces feta cheese, crumbled
4 ounces cream cheese, softened
½ cup ricotta cheese
1 teaspoon fresh lemon
¼ teaspoon cumin
Pinch of nutmeg
6 6-inch whole-wheat tortillas
Salt and pepper to taste

Directions

Place olive oil in a large pan on medium heat. Sauté onion until golden. Add garlic and spinach, and cook, stirring, until spinach begins to wilt. Drain onion and spinach on paper towels. In a medium bowl, mix the feta cheese, cream cheese, ricotta cheese, and seasonings. Fold into the spinach mixture. Spoon ¼ of mixture onto the center of each tortilla. Roll tortilla up, enchilada-style, and bake at 350 degrees for 10–15 minutes, until cooked through.

Yield: Serves 6.

Nutrition information per serving: Calories: 197; Fat: 13g; Carbohydrates: 19g; Fiber: 2g; Protein: 10g.

❖ Grilled Portobello
Sandwiches with Goat Cheese

Ingredients
1 red pepper
1 tablespoon olive oil
1 tablespoon balsamic vinegar
Dash of salt and pepper
2 large portobello mushroom caps
2 ounces goat cheese, crumbled
½ recipe of Italian garlic bread (4 slices), see page 229
5 large lettuce leaves

Directions
Cut off the top and bottom of the red pepper. Slice off all four sides and discard the core. Combine olive oil, balsamic vinegar, salt and pepper in a small bowl. Take the four slices of the red pepper and dip in the vinaigrette. Brush remaining oil and vinegar onto portobello caps. Place vegetables on grill for 5–8 minutes, flipping once, and cooking until brown (do not burn). You can also roast the vegetables in a 450-degree oven for 5–10 minutes, flipping once. Prepare Italian garlic bread. Layer red pepper and portobellos on garlic bread and top with goat cheese and lettuce, followed by the top slice of bread. Serve immediately.

Yield: 2 sandwiches.

Nutrition information per serving: Calories: 550; Fat: 29g; Carbohydrates: 44g; Fiber: 6g; Protein: 20g.

VEGETABLES/SIDES

❖ Guacamole*

Ingredients
2 ripe avocados
½ teaspoon garlic powder
¼ teaspoon cayenne pepper
1 medium ripe tomato, seeded and chopped
Juice of half a lime
Salt and pepper to taste

Directions
Check the ripeness of the avocados. The skin should be dark green to black, and the avocado should give slightly to the touch. Halve the avocados, remove the pits, and spoon fruit into a bowl. Mash with a fork until soft. Blend in garlic powder and cayenne pepper. Add salt and pepper to taste. Stir in lime juice. Top with diced tomatoes. Place avocado pit back in guacamole until ready to serve. This will keep the avocado from turning brown. Serve with fresh veggies, warm tortillas, or tortilla chips.

Yield: Serves 4.

Nutrition information per serving: Calories: 169; Fat: 16g; Carbohydrates: 9g; Fiber: 5g; Protein: 5g.

❖ Summer Salsa*

Ingredients
6 medium tomatoes, seeded
½ teaspoon salt
½ red onion, chopped
½ cup celery, finely diced
½ cup cucumber, finely diced
1 small, sweet banana pepper, chopped
½ cup mango, diced in small squares
Juice of one lime
½ teaspoon garlic powder
Salt and cayenne pepper to taste

Directions

Dice tomatoes and spread on paper towels to drain. Sprinkle with ½ tea-spoon salt. After 30 minutes, place tomatoes in a serving bowl. Add chopped vegetables and stir until well combined. Allow to sit at least one hour. You can also blend the salsa in the food processor for a smoother consistency.

Yield: Serves 4.

Nutrition information per serving: Calories: 70; Fat: 1g; Carbohydrates: 25g; Fiber: 4g; Protein: 2g.

❖ Tasty Green Beans*

Ingredients
1 pound green beans, washed
½ cup red onion, thinly sliced

DRESSING
1 tablespoon water
2 tablespoons soy sauce
3 tablespoons rice vinegar
1 tablespoon sesame oil
2 teaspoons fresh ginger, minced
1½ tablespoons dry mustard powder
1 teaspoon garlic powder

Directions

Trim the green beans and cut into pieces that are about 1 inch long. Boil two cups water, and then add green beans when water comes to a roll-ing boil. Prepare a large bowl of ice water while beans are cooking. Cook green beans for 3–5 minutes until crisp-tender. With a slotted spoon, spoon beans into the ice water to stop the cooking. After several minutes, drain beans in a colander. In a large bowl, combine water, soy sauce, vine-gar, and oil. Whisk ingredients until well blended. Add ginger. Stir in dry mustard and garlic powder. Toss the green beans with the red onion and dressing.

Yield: Serves 4.

Nutrition information per serving: Calories: 52; Fat: 3g; Carbohydrates: 4g; Fiber: 2g; Protein: 2g.

❖ Broccoli Rabe with Garlic and Pine Nuts*

Ingredients
1 tablespoon olive oil
8–10 stalks rapini
1 tablespoon soy sauce
2 cloves garlic, minced
2 tablespoons pine nuts
Salt and pepper to taste

Directions
Cut rapini about midway through the stalks. Chop the leaves and florets into large bite-sized pieces. Heat olive oil in sauté pan on medium-high heat. Sauté rapini with garlic and soy sauce for several minutes, until slightly wilted. Toss in pine nuts and stir. Add salt and pepper to taste. This tastes great tossed with fettuccini.

Yield: Serves 4.

Nutrition information per serving: Calories: 70; Fat: 5g; Carbohydrates: 4g; Fiber: <1g; Protein: 3g.

❖ Sautéed Kale with Feta*

Ingredients
1 large bunch kale, about 6–8 stalks
1 tablespoon olive oil
4 ounces feta cheese
Salt and pepper to taste

Directions
Tear leaves off kale stalks and discard the stalks. Chop the leaves into large pieces. Heat oil in a large sauté pan. Add kale and stir-fry for several minutes until wilted. Remove from heat and place in serving bowl. Toss kale with feta cheese, salt and pepper. Serve tossed with pasta, lemon juice and olive oil or as a side dish.

Yield: Serves 4.

Nutrition information per serving: Calories: 105; Fat: 9g; Carbohydrates: 1g; Fiber: 0g; Protein: 4g.

❖ Dharma's Collard Greens*

Ingredients
4 cups collard greens, washed
1 tablespoon brown sugar
1 tablespoon olive oil
1 teaspoon onion powder
Salt and pepper (to taste)

Directions
Add oil to a large saucepan. Add ¼ cup water to pan and heat on medium-high until boiling. Tear collard green leaves off the stalks. Chop leaves into large strips. Heat collard greens in water until soft and dark green. Stir in brown sugar; add onion powder, salt and pepper to taste. You can also season with 2 tablespoons vinegar or hot sauce.

Yield: Serves 4.

Nutrition information per serving: Calories: 25; Fat: <1g; Carbohydrates: 6g; Fiber: 1g; Protein: 1g.

❖ Baked Peas with Cheese*

Ingredients
2 15-ounce cans green peas, drained
1 10-ounce can low-fat cream of mushroom soup
1 8-ounce can water chestnuts, sliced
6 ounces sharp cheddar cheese, grated
Salt and pepper to taste

Directions
Add peas, mushroom soup, and water chestnuts to a large casserole dish. Stir in 4 ounces of cheese and add salt and pepper. Mix well and top with remaining cheese. Bake, uncovered, at 350 degrees for 30 minutes.

Yield: Serves 8.

Nutrition information per serving: Calories: 170; Fat: 8g; Carbohydrates: 15g; Fiber: 4g; Protein: 9g.

❖ Lemon-Ginger Carrots*

Ingredients
2 cups baby carrots, halved
1 tablespoon butter
Juice of one lemon
1 teaspoon fresh ginger, minced
Salt to taste

Directions
Heat 2 cups of water to boiling. Add baby carrots to water and cover. Steam for 5–10 minutes, until soft. In a separate small pot, heat butter and ginger on medium heat for 2 minutes, until ginger starts to turn golden brown. Add steamed carrots, lemon juice, and salt to taste. Stir gently and serve warm.

Yield: Serves 4.

Nutrition information per serving: Calories: 76; Fat: 3g; Carbohydrates: 10g; Fiber: 2g; Protein: 1g.

❖ Roasted Sweet Potatoes and Winter Squash with Rosemary

Ingredients
2 medium sweet potatoes
4 cups winter squash (acorn or butternut)
2 tablespoons fresh rosemary
2 tablespoons olive oil
½ teaspoon oregano
1 teaspoon garlic powder
1 teaspoon onion powder
Salt and pepper to taste

Directions
Heat oven to 375 degrees. Wash and peel potatoes. Halve the winter squash. Cook vegetables for 20–25 minutes, until they begin to soften. Set aside to cool. After they cool, scoop out the flesh of the winter squash. Cut into two-inch squares. Cut sweet potatoes into two-inch squares as well. Combine herbs, oil, and seasonings in small bowl. Whisk until well blended. In an large oiled baking dish, place potatoes and winter squash side by side in a single layer. Spoon seasoning over vegetables. Bake for 20–30 minutes until cooked through and soft.

Yield: Serves 4.

Nutrition information per serving: Calories: 190; Fat: 7g; Carbohydrates: 32g; Fiber: 4g; Protein: 3g.

❖ Healthy Fries

Ingredients
3 large potatoes
1 tablespoon olive oil
Salt to taste

Directions
Slice potatoes into shoestring or steak-fry thickness. Pour olive oil and salt over potatoes, and stir until coated. Spread potatoes on large baking sheet

in a single layer. Cook for 30 minutes at 375 degrees. Flip potatoes once, and cook for an additional 10–15 minutes until golden and crispy.

Yield: Serves 6.

Nutrition information per serving: Calories: 162; Fat: 2g; Carbohydrates: 32g; Fiber: 4g; Protein: 4g.

❖ Barbecued Tofu*

Ingredients
16 ounce block of extra-firm tofu
2 tablespoons olive oil
⅔ cup barbecue sauce
1 tablespoon honey
1 teaspoon garlic powder
½ teaspoon salt

Directions
Slice tofu into small rectangles, about 1 inch wide, 2 inches long, and ½ inch thick. Heat oil in a large sauté pan on medium-high heat. Place tofu in a single layer in the pan. Cook for 4–5 minutes until underside is golden brown. Flip tofu and cook an additional 3–4 minutes until both sides are golden brown. Turn heat to medium-low. Drizzle honey and barbecue sauce over tofu. Sprinkle with garlic powder and salt. Cover and let tofu steam in the sauce for several minutes.

Yield: Serves 4.

Nutrition information per serving: Calories: 220; Fat: 15g; Carbohydrates: 11g; Fiber: 2g; Protein: 13g.

❖ Soy Sausage Balls*

Ingredients
1 14-ounce roll of soy sausage
1 8-ounce package sharp cheddar cheese (or soy cheddar cheese)
1¾ cups baking mix
¼ cup olive oil

Directions
Shred cheddar cheese. Put soy sausage, cheddar cheese, baking mix, and olive oil in a large mixing bowl. Knead ingredients with hands until mixture is fully blended. Make small balls of mixture and place on a baking sheet. Put the baking sheet in the freezer for 6 to 8 hours. Take the frozen sausage balls and place in a zipper freezer bag. Freeze the balls to use as desired. To serve, take out the balls you wish to serve and place on a lightly greased baking sheet. Spray balls with olive oil Pam. Bake at 350 degrees for 10–15 minutes, until cooked through and golden brown.

Yield: Makes 90 balls.

Nutrition information per serving: Calories (per soy sausage ball): 30; Fat: 2g; Carbohydrates: 2g; Fiber: <1g; Protein: 1g.

DESSERTS

❖ Pineapple Upside-Down Cake

Ingredients
1 cup pastry flour
1 teaspoon baking powder
½ teaspoon salt
¼ cup butter
½ cup pecans, chopped finely
¾ cup brown sugar
1 fresh pineapple, peeled, cored, sliced in ½-inch slices
3 eggs
¾ cup sugar
⅓ cup pineapple juice
Maraschino cherries for topping

Directions

Preheat oven to 350 degrees. Combine flour, baking powder, and salt in medium bowl. Set aside. In a large cast-iron skillet, melt butter over medium-low heat. Add pecans and brown sugar and stir well, then remove from heat. Place pineapple slices over this mixture, overlapping as little as possible. Separate egg yolks from egg whites and set the egg whites aside. Pour yolks into a large mixing bowl, and mix well. Add the sugar in parts, stirring well. Pour flour mixture into the egg yolks and stir. Stir in the pineapple juice. In a separate small mixing bowl, beat the egg whites until peaks are formed, and whites become stiff. Gently fold egg whites into the large bowl with the rest of the ingredients. Gently pour this batter into the skillet, over the pineapple rings. Place the skillet in the oven and cook at 350 degrees for 40 minutes, or until inserted toothpick comes out clean. After cooking, remove skillet from oven and let cool. Invert the pineapple upside-down cake onto a large serving plate, and garnish with maraschino cherries.

Yield: Serves 10.

Nutrition information per serving: Calories: 302; Fat: 11g; Carbohydrates: 51g; Fiber: 1g; Protein: 4g.

❖ Healthy Carrot Cake

Ingredients

2½ cups all-purpose flour
2 teaspoons baking soda
1 teaspoon cinnamon
½ teaspoon fresh ground nutmeg
2 cups carrots, finely grated
¼ cup orange juice (fresh squeezed, if possible)
1 tablespoon vanilla
¼ cup canola oil
½ cup brown sugar
¼ cup applesauce
½ cup fresh pineapple,
    chopped in small pieces

LEMON-WALNUT FROSTING
4 ounces low-fat cream cheese, softened
2 tablespoons butter, softened
4 cups powdered sugar
1 teaspoon vanilla
Juice from one lemon
½ cup walnuts, finely chopped

Directions
Preheat oven to 350 degrees. Sift flour, baking soda, cinnamon, and nut-meg together in a medium bowl. Mix well. In a separate large mixing bowl, place carrots, orange juice, vanilla, oil, brown sugar, and fruit. Stir mixture until well combined. Add the dry ingredients in parts, and mix well. Pour batter into a large cake pan and cook for 45 minutes. Cake is done when inserted toothpick comes out clean.

For frosting, mix together cream cheese and butter in a medium bowl. Add powdered sugar in parts and mix. Add vanilla and lemon juice. When cake is cool, spread icing on cake; sprinkle walnuts on top.

Yield: Serves 16.

Nutrition information per serving: Calories: 305; Fat: 9g; Carbohydrates: 54g; Fiber: 1g; Protein: 4g.

❖ Tasty Tofu Cake

Ingredients
Butter and flour for cake pan
2¼ cups pastry flour
2 teaspoons baking powder
½ teaspoon salt
8 ounces soft or silken tofu
1 cup low-fat milk
½ cup applesauce
½ cup butter
1 cup sugar
¼ cup brown sugar
2 teaspoons vanilla

STRAWBERRY PECAN ICING

8 ounces low-fat cream cheese, softened
2 tablespoons butter, softened
1 teaspoon vanilla
½ cup fresh strawberries, mashed
4 cups sifted powdered sugar
½ cup pecans, finely chopped

Directions

Preheat oven to 350 degrees. Grease and flour a large cake pan or muffin tin. Or, place muffin cups in muffin tin. Place flour, baking powder, and salt in a small bowl. Place tofu, milk, and applesauce in a blender or large food processor, and blend until smooth. In a large mixing bowl, beat butter, sugar, and brown sugar until well blended. Add tofu mixture to the butter and sugar. Mix well. Add dry ingredients in parts and blend. Add vanilla and stir. Pour cake batter into the pan or muffin tins. Bake for 30 minutes, until inserted toothpick comes out clean.

While cake is cooking, cream together cream cheese and butter. Add vanilla and strawberries; stir. Slowly add the powdered sugar in parts, and blend to your desired consistency. Spread onto cooled cake, and sprinkle with pecans.

Yield: Serves 20.

Nutrition information per serving: Calories: 310; Fat: 11g; Carbohydrates: 53g; Fiber: 1g; Protein: 4g.

❖ Nut Meringue Cookies*

Ingredients

4 large egg whites
¼ teaspoon salt
¼ teaspoon cream of tartar
1 teaspoon vanilla
1 cup sugar
1 cup chopped walnuts, pecans,
   and/or almonds

Directions

Beat egg whites, salt, cream of tartar, and vanilla until peaks form. Gradually add sugar and beat until peaks are stiff. Fold in nuts. Cover cookie sheet with wax paper, parchment paper, or a paper bag. Drop batter by tablespoons onto the paper. Bake at 225 degrees for 2–3 hours, depending on indoor humidity.

Yield: 40 cookies.

Nutrition information per serving: Calories: 40; Fat: 2g; Carbohydrates: 5g; Fiber: <1g; Protein: 2g.

The Pain-Free Back Exercises

Use the following exercises with Step 1, the Pain-Free Back Exercise Program. Begin gentle stretching exercises daily, including the exercises discussed below. As your acute back pain symptoms are under control, start the range-of-motion exercises described on page 262. Follow with the other exercises to strengthen the muscles and support the back.

Stretching Exercises

Stretch throughout the day to keep muscles limber and flexible. Stretching helps to ease stiffness and allows you to be more active throughout the day.

Chest and Mid-Back
Place a broom handle or a long pole behind your back and across your shoulders with your hands supporting the long handle or pole at each end. Then slowly rotate your torso to the left; repeat this movement in the opposite direction (figure A.1).

Shoulders
Hold a broom handle or long pole with both hands over your head and slowly stretch from side to side like a pendulum several times. Then place the pole at shoulder level in front of you and gently turn to the right as far as is comfortable, then to the left. Repeat several times (figure A.2).

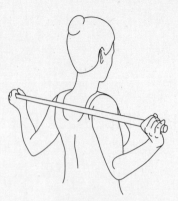

Figure A.1

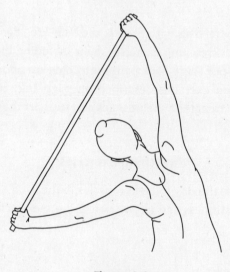

Figure A.2

Neck

Place one hand on the side of your head just above the ear and gently push as if you were trying to place your other ear to your shoulder. Gradually build pressure but do not force the movement. Hold and then relax (figure A.3).

Legs and Hamstrings

Stand upright and put foot on bench (or step). Slowly bend forward at the hip while keeping your back straight. Alternate to the other leg and repeat exercise. You should feel the stretch behind your thigh (figure A.4).

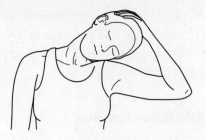

Figure A.3

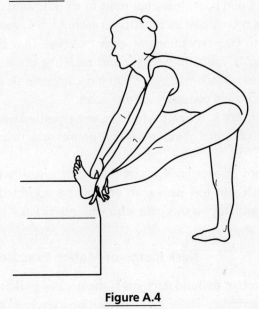

Figure A.4

Back

This exercise will help keep your posture straight and alleviate stress on the back and hips. Lie on your back with your knees bent and feet flat on

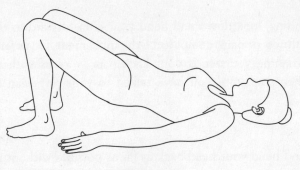

Figure A.5

the floor, hip-width apart. While contracting your abdominal muscles, press your lower back against the floor. You will feel your pelvis rock (tilt) toward your shoulders. The bottom of your buttocks and your pelvis will come slightly off the floor during the action (figure A.5).

Range-of-Motion Exercises

These exercises are designed to build flexibility and strength in the neck, shoulders, and back. It is important to work toward a goal of doing these exercises twice a day, 20 repetitions each. At first, you may only be able to do one to two repetitions of each exercise. That is a reasonable start. However, as you gain strength and mobility, move into twice-daily, 20 repetitions of each routine. If you have any pain or unusual feeling, stop the exercise and contact your physician.

Sometimes it is helpful to have some gentle assistance from a family member or friend. Your physician or physical therapist can show you how.

A word of caution: Do not hold your breath while performing any exercise. If you feel pain with any of the suggested exercises, stop the exercise and discuss this pain with your physician.

Neck Range-of-Motion Exercises

It is important to build strength in the neck as well as improve the mobility and flexibility. These range-of-motion exercises will enable your body to perform more effectively. While flexion should be done standing, the rest of the neck exercises can be performed sitting or standing, whichever is more comfortable for you.

Flexion

While standing, look down and bend your chin forward to the chest. If you feel stiffness or pain, do not force the movement. Go as far as you can without straining yourself. If your back pain worsens with this or any exercise then stop until you have talked to your physician or physical therapist.

Extension

Look up and bend your head back as far as possible without forcing any movement.

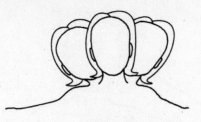

Figure A.6

Lateral flexion

Lateral Flexion

Tilt your left ear to your left shoulder (but do not raise the shoulder). If you feel pain or resistance, do not force the motion.

Now tilt the right ear to the right shoulder just as you did for the left ear (figure A.6).

Rotation

Turn to look over your left shoulder. Try to make your chin even with your shoulder. Go as far as is comfortable, but do not force the movement.

Now turn and look over your right shoulder, as you did with the left.

Neck Isometric Exercises

Neck isometric exercises are more advanced exercises to help strengthen the muscles of the neck. Try these gently and gradually after the range of motion of your neck is improved as much as possible. Again, do not hold your breath.

Isometric Flexion

Place hand on your forehead. Try to look down while resisting the motion with your hand. Hold for 6 seconds. Count out loud.

Place your hands on the back of your head. Try to look up and back while resisting the motion with your hands. Hold for 6 seconds. Count out loud.

Isometric Lateral Flexion

Start with your head straight. Place your left hand just above your left ear (figure A.7). Try to tilt your head to the left but resist the motion with your left hand. Hold for 6 seconds. Count out loud.

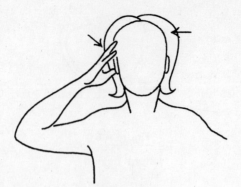

Figure A.7

Isometric lateral flexion

Now place your right hand just above your right ear. Try to tilt your head to the right but resist the movement with your right hand. Hold for 6 seconds. Count out loud.

Isometric Rotation

Place your left hand above your ear and near your left forehead. Now try to look over your left shoulder, but resist the motion with your left hand. The hand should not be placed on the jaw. Hold for 6 seconds. Count out loud.

Now place your right hand above your ear and near your right forehead. Now try to look over your right shoulder but resist the motion with your right hand. Hold for 6 seconds. Count out loud.

Shoulder Range-of-Motion Exercises

The following five range-of-motion exercises will increase the flexibility of the shoulders and arms. Increasing the number of exercises can increase the strength of the arms.

Shoulder External Rotation

This exercise increases the motion you use to comb your hair. You may sit, stand, or lie down to do these exercises.

Clasp your hands behind your head. Pull your elbows together until they are as close as possible in front of your chin. Separate the elbows to the side as much as possible.

Repeat this, gradually increasing to 5, then 10, then up to 20 repetitions. Repeat these 2 or 3 times daily.

Shoulder Internal Rotation

Shoulder internal rotation increases the flexibility of the shoulders. Using the same motions women use to fasten a bra in the back or men use to put a wallet in a back pocket, move your arms in the position as shown in figure A.8. This exercise is best done standing and is often done in the shower using a washcloth to wash your upper back or a towel to dry it.

Put your hand behind your back. Then put the other hand behind your back and cross your wrists as shown in the picture. Return the hands to rest at your side.

Repeat, gradually increasing to 5, then 10, then up to 20 repetitions. Repeat twice daily.

Shoulder Flexion

Shoulder flexion holds both arms down at your sides. Raise the left arm straight up and reach overhead toward the ceiling. Now do the same with

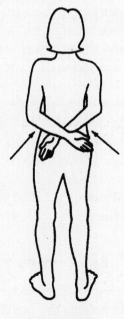

Figure A.8

Shoulder internal rotation

the right arm. Continue this motion as you alternate left-right-left-right. Gradually increase to 5, then 10, then up to 20 repetitions, and repeat the exercise twice daily.

Shoulder Abduction

Raise both arms straight out away from your sides, then raise each arm overhead toward the ceiling and up above your head. Do this with your palm up or palm down.

If this exercise is painful while sitting or standing, you can also do it while lying on your bed. Use a stick (a broom handle will do) as you raise your arms, hold the stick with both hands and keep the arms straight, up over your head as far as possible. The strength of the less painful arm will help the painful arm move more easily.

Repeat this, gradually increasing to 5, then 10, then 20 repetitions two or three times a day.

Once you have mastered the exercise, go to the second part. This involves raising your arms out to the side, one at a time, then slowly making big circles.

Repeat this, gradually increasing to 5, then 10, then 20 repetitions two or three times a day.

Shoulder Girdle Rotation

This exercise can be done in a sitting or standing position and is fun to do during the day to relieve neck and shoulder tension and maintain shoulder girdle flexibility.

Roll shoulders in a forward circle; raise shoulders toward the ears in a shrugging motion. Roll shoulders back and chest out as in a military stance. Lower the shoulders and bring them forward. Think of it as a simple shoulder roll in a circle. Now reverse the process, rolling your shoulder girdle in a backwards circle.

Repeat this, gradually increasing to 5, then 10, then 20 repetitions two or three times a day if possible.

Back Exercises

As you do the following strengthening exercises, it is very important that you breathe properly while holding the position. Counting to six aloud will enable you to do this easily. If you experience shortness of breath, stop and talk to your doctor or physical therapist.

Cheek to Cheek

This is a convenient exercise because you can do it anywhere, anytime, and practically in any position. It strengthens the muscles of the buttocks that help support the back and the legs. When sitting, you will actually raise up out of the chair because of the contraction of the muscle groups in the buttocks.

Press your buttocks together and hold for a 6-second count. Relax and repeat. Gradually increase up to 5, then 10, then 20 repetitions. Repeat two times daily. Do this exercise frequently during the day.

Pelvic Tilt

This is one of the best exercises you can do to strengthen your abdominal muscles, which in turn help support your back. It will also help tone your stomach muscles. Do this exercise lying on your back in bed or on the floor, whichever is more comfortable.

Relax and raise your arms above your head. Keep your knees bent. Now comes the tricky part! Tighten the muscles of your lower abdomen and your buttocks at the same time to flatten your back against the floor or bed. Hold the flat-back position for a 6-second count. Now relax.

Repeat this exercise 2 or 3 times to start and gradually increase to 5, then 10, then 20 repetitions.

If you have trouble, contact your physical therapist or physician and have him or her demonstrate the exercise. This may be particularly necessary if you want to do this exercise standing up or sitting in a chair.

Bridging

This exercise strengthens the muscles in the back. Lie on your back on the floor or in bed and bend (flex) your hips and knees (figure A.9). Now lift your hips and buttocks off the bed or floor 4 to 6 inches, forcing the small

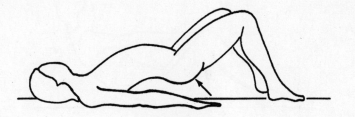

Figure A.9

A bridging exercise

of the back out flat; and tighten the buttock and hip muscles to maintain this position. Hold this position for a count of six seconds. Now, relax and lower your hips and buttocks to the floor or bed.

Repeat this exercise, gradually increasing to 5, then 10, then 20 repetitions as tolerated. Repeat twice daily if possible.

Partial Sit-Up

This is one of the more vigorous exercises. Its purpose is to build abdominal strength to give the back greater support.

To do this exercise lie on back on your bed or on the floor, whichever is more comfortable, with your knees bent (see figure A.10).

Raise your head and shoulder blades off the floor or bed. Hold that position for a 6-second count. Slowly return to the beginning position of lying on your back.

Start this exercise slowly with 1 or 2 repetitions until your body adjusts. Gradually increase to 5, then 10 repetitions.

Back Extension

For this exercise to strengthen the back muscles, lie on your bed or on the floor in a prone (stomach-down) position. A pillow may be used under the stomach to help make this position more comfortable.

Raise your head, arms, and legs off the floor. Do not bend your knees. This must be done with your body straight in extension. Hold for six seconds while you count out loud. Relax and repeat.

Gradually increase up to 5, then 10 repetitions. If you experience discomfort, check with your physician or physical therapist before you continue.

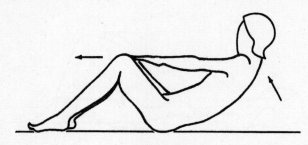

Figure A.10

A partial sit-up exercise

Cat Camel

Do not do this exercise if you have very painful knees, ankles, or hands because it places pressure on these areas.

The position for this exercise is a crawling position (figure A.11). Hands must be directly under your shoulders. Take a deep breath and arch your back as a frightened cat does, lowering your head. Hold that position while you count the 6 seconds out loud. Now exhale and drop the arched back slowly, raising your head.

Start this exercise slowly with one or two repetitions. Increase up to 5, and then 10 repetitions if possible.

Wall Push

This exercise is good for the back because it encourages the body's extension positions.

Stand spread-eagle with your back against a solid wall. Now arch your back inward slowly so your shoulders touch the wall.

Gradually increase repetitions from 1 to 5 or more. This exercise is fun because you can do it any time you feel you need a good body stretch. Repeat two times daily.

Back Flexibility

Lie on your back on the floor with knees bent and feet flat on the floor. Raise hands toward the ceiling. Now move arms and turn the head to the right, while the knees move to the left. Reverse the above, then repeat. Gradually increase up to 5, and then 10 repetitions daily.

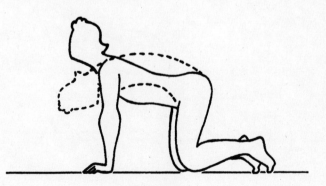

Figure A.11

Cat camel exercise

Bicycling

Lying on your back, move your feet and legs in the air as if you were riding a bicycle. Count to 6, and relax. Repeat and gradually increase to 5, then 10 repetitions once or twice daily if tolerated.

Hip Exercises

These exercises are good not only for the hips but for the back and the knees.

Flexion

You can do these exercises on the floor or in bed, but don't do them if you have had a hip or knee total joint replacement.

Bend the left knee to the chest, and then bend the right knee to the chest. If needed, you can help by using your hands to help bend the knee. Repeat, alternating left and right knees. Try to increase to five, then 10, then up to 20 repetitions, twice daily.

Pull both knees to the chest at the same time (figure A.12). Hold this position for six seconds and then slowly rock from side to side while holding the knees. Gently let your legs down. Repeat, gradually increasing to 5, then 10, then 20 repetitions, twice daily.

Abduction

This can be done lying on the floor or in bed. While lying on your back slide your left leg out to the side, with knee straight or slightly bent, then

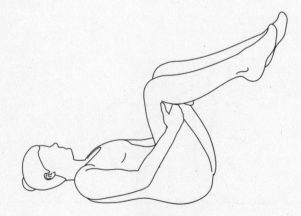

Figure A.12

Hip flexion

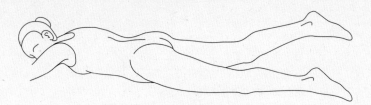

Figure A.13

Hip extension

return to the starting position. Now do the same movement with the right leg. Gradually increase to 5, then 10, then 20 repetitions for each leg, twice daily.

Extension

This can be done lying on your stomach on the floor or in bed. Keeping your knee straight, lift your left thigh straight up off the floor about eight inches (figure A.13). Hold this position while you count to six. Repeat with the right leg, then alternate legs, and gradually increase to 5, then 10, then 20 repetitions, twice daily. If there is severe pain, stop until you talk to your doctor.

Rotation

Lie on your back on the floor or in bed. With your knees straight, turn your knees in and touch the toes of your feet together. Now turn the knees out. Repeat this, gradually increasing to 5, then 10, then 20 repetitions, twice daily.

Knee and Leg Exercises

Extension

This exercise can strengthen the muscles of the thighs (quadriceps muscles), which offer a major support for the knee. You can do this while reading, watching television, or riding in an airplane. The more you do it, the stronger the support for your knees.

While sitting in a chair, support your leg on a chair or table and straighten your knee as much as possible (figure A.14). Then tighten your kneecap (push the knee down) until you feel the muscles of the thigh tighten. Keep that muscle tight and count to six. Relax, then repeat, gradually increasing to 5, then 10, then 15 repetitions, twice daily.

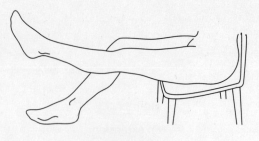

Figure A.14

Knee and leg extension

Straight Leg Raise

While lying on the floor on in bed, bend your knee slightly as shown (figure A.15), or bend one knee to the chest if you have chronic back pain. Raise the other leg slowly while keeping the back firmly on the floor or bed. Raise your leg as high as you can, but stop if your back begins to arch. Hold and count to six. Lower your leg, and then repeat the stops for the opposite leg. Repeat for both legs, gradually increasing to 5, then 10, then 20 repetitions, twice daily. If you have severe pain with this or any exercise, stop immediately and talk to your doctor.

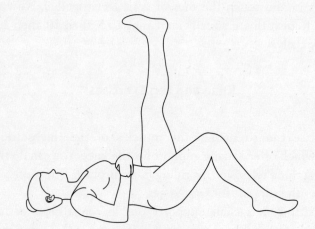

Figure A.15

Straight leg raise

Flexion
You can do this on the floor or in bed. Lie on your stomach and bend your knees as far as you can toward your back. Straighten your knee, then repeat, gradually increasing to 5, then 10, then 20 repetitions, twice daily.

Ankle and Foot Exercise

This exercise is easy to do and can be performed while seated almost anywhere. Raise your toes as high as you can with your heels on the floor (figure A.16). Then press your toes to the floor and raise the heels as high as you can see. Finally, rotate the ankles in a circle. Repeat, gradually increasing to 5, then 10, then 20 repetitions, twice daily.

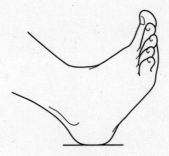

Figure A.16

Ankle and foot exercise

Resources

Pain-Related Organizations

American Academy of Medical
Acupuncture (AAMA)
4929 Wilshire Boulevard, Suite 428
Los Angeles, CA 90010
323-937-5514

American Academy of Pain
Management
13947 Mono Way, #A
Sonora, CA 95370
209-533-9744

American Chronic Pain Association
P.O. Box 850
Rocklin, CA 95677
916-632-0922

American Fibromyalgia Syndrome
Association
6380 E. Tanque Verde, Suite D
Tucson, AZ 85715
520-733-1570

American Pain Foundation
201 N. Charles Street, Suite 710
Baltimore, MD 21201-4111
888-614-PAIN (7246)

American Pain Society
4700 W. Lake Ave.
Glenview, IL 60025
847-375-4715

Arthritis Foundation
1314 Spring Street
Atlanta, GA 30309
800-283-7800; 404-872-7100

Arthritis Society
250 Floor Street East, Suite 901
Toronto, Ontario
Canada M4W 3P2
416-967-1414

Fibromyalgia Association
P.O. Box 21988
Columbus, OH 43221-0988
614-457-4222 (phone);
614-457-2729 (fax)

Fibromyalgia Network
5700 Stockdale Highway, Suite 100
Bakersfield, CA 93309
805-631-1950

North American Spine Society
22 Calendar Court, 2nd Floor
LaGrange, IL 60525
E-mail: info@spine.org

Spondylitis Association of America
14827 Ventura Blvd., #222
Sherman Oaks, CA 91403
800-777-8189

Websites

The following websites offer self-help products for those with chronic
pain and back problems:

Accessibility Products Online
http://www.accesstoday.com

ADI Assistive Devices
http://www.geocel.com/adi/
    home.htm

Aids for Arthritis
http://www.aidsforarthritis.com

Comfort-Discovered
http://e-bility.com/
    comfort-discovered/arthritis.php

Dynamic Living
http://www.dynamic-living.com/
    alternatives.htm

Independent Living Products
http://www.ilp-online.com

Keyless Keyboards
http://www.keybowl.com

Life with Ease
http://www.lifewithease.com

Maddak, Inc.
http://www.maddak.com

Maxi Aids
http://www.maxiaids.com

North Coast Medical
http://www.ncmedical.com

Products for Seniors
http://www.productsforseniors.
    com/arthritis_aids.htm

Sammons Preston
http://www.sammonspreston.com

The Boulevard
http://www.blvd.com

References and
Supporting Research

Akhondzadeh, S., L. Kashani, M. Mobaseri, et al. "Passionflower in the treatment of opiates withdrawal: A double-blind randomized controlled trial." *Journal of Clinical Pharmacy and Therapeutics* 26 (2001): 369–73.

Andersson, G. B., T. Lucente, A. M. Davis, et al. "A comparison of osteopathic spinal manipulation with standard care for patients with low back pain." *New England Journal of Medicine* 341 (1999): 1426–31.

Belch, J. J., et al. "Evening primrose oil and borage oil in rheumatologic conditions." *American Journal of Clinical Nutrition* 71 (2000) (1 Supplement): 352S–565.

Benson, H., et al. "Relaxation Response: Bridge between psychiatry and medicine." *Medical Clinics of North America* 61 (1977): 929–38.

Bigos, S., O. Bowyer, G. Braen, et al. "Acute low back problems in adults." Rockville, Md.: U.S. Department of Health and Human Services, Agency for Health Care Policy and Research Pub. no. 95-0643, December 1994.

Brady, L. H., K. Henry, J. F. Luth II, et al. "The effects of shiatsu on lower back pain." *Journal of Holistic Nursing* 19 (2000): 57–70.

Castleman, M. *The Healing Herbs: The Ultimate Guide to the Curative Power of Nature's Medicines.* New York: Bantam Books, 1995, 27.

Cherkin, D. C., R. A. Deyo, M. Battie, et al. "A comparison of physical therapy, chiropractic manipulation, and provision of an educational booklet for the treatment of patients with low back pain." *New England Journal of Medicine,* 339 (Oct. 1998): 1021–29.

Chrubasik, S., E. Eisenberg, E. Balan, et al. "Treatment of low back pain exacerbations with willow bark extract: A randomized double-blind study." *American Journal of Medicine* 109 (2000): 9–14.

Dulloo, A. G., C. Duret, D. Rohrer, et al. "Efficacy of a green tea extract rich in catechin polyphenols and caffeine in increasing 24-hour energy expenditure and fat oxidation in humans." *American Journal of Clinical Nutrition* 70 (1999): 1040–41.

Elkayam, O., S. Ben Itzhak, E. Avrahami, et al. "Multidisciplinary approach to chronic back pain: prognostic elements of the outcome." *Clinical and Experimental Rheumatology* 14 (May–June 1996): 281–88.

Epel, E. S., et al. "Stress and body shape: Stress-induced cortisol secretion is consistently greater among women with central fat." *Psychosomatic Medicine* 62 (Sept.–Oct. 2000): 623–32.

Fiechtner, J. J., and R. R. Brodeur. "Manual and manipulation techniques for rheumatic disease." *Medical Clinics of North America* 86 (Jan. 2002): 91–103.

Ghoname, E. A., W. F. Craig, P. F. White, et al. "Percutaneous electrical nerve stimulation for low back pain: A randomized crossover study." *Journal of the American Medical Association* 281 (19) (1999): 1795.

Gura, S. T. "Yoga for stress reduction and injury prevention at work." *Work* 19 (2002): 3–7.

Han, T. S., J. S. Schouten, M. E. Lean, et al. "The prevalence of low back pain and associations with body fatness, fat distribution and height." *International Journal of Obesity and Related Metabolic Disorders* 21 (July 1997): 600–607.

Han, T. S., M. A. Tijhuis, M. E. Lean, et al. "Quality of life in relation to overweight and body fat distribution." *American Journal of Public Health* 88 (1998): 1814–20.

Hegarty, V., H. May, K. Khaw. "Tea drinking and bone mineral density in older women." *American Journal of Clinical Nutrition* 71 (2000): 1003–7.

Hernandez-Reif, M., T. Field, J. Krasnegor, et al. "Lower back pain is reduced and range of motion increased after massage therapy." *International Journal of Neuroscience* 106 (2001): 131–45.

Kim, H., K. Son, H. Chang, et al. "Inhibition of rat adjuvant-induced arthritis by ginkgetin, a biflavone from Ginkgo biloba leaves." *Planta Medica* 54 (1999): 465–67.

Layman, D., R. Boileau, D. Erickson, et al. "A reduced ratio of dietary carbohydrate to protein improves body composition and blood lipid profiles during weight loss in adult women." *Journal of Nutrition* 133 (2003): 411–17.

McAlindon, T. E., M. P. LaValley, J. P. Gulin, et al. "Glucosamine and chondroitin for treatment of osteoarthritis: A systematic quality assessment and meta-analysis." *Journal of the American Medical Association* 283 (2000): 1469–75.

Rooks, D. S., et al. "The effects of progressive strength training and aerobic exercise on muscle strength and cardiovascular fitness in women with fibromyalgia: A pilot study." *Arthritis and Rheumatism* 47 (Feb. 2000): 22–28.

Agency for Healthcare Research and Quality. "S-adenosyl-l-methionine for treatment of depression, osteoarthritis, and liver disease." Publication no. 02-E033, August 2002, Rockville, Md.

Schrader, E. "Equivalence of a St. John's wort extract (Ze 117) and fluoxetine: A randomized, controlled study in mild-moderate depression." *International Clinical Psychopharmacology* 15 (2000): 61–68.

Sondike, S. B., N. M. Copperman, M. S. Jacobson. "Low-carbohydrate dieting increases weight loss but not cardiovascular risk in obese adolescents: A randomized controlled trial." *Journal of Adolescent Health* 26 (2000): 91.

Toda, T., N. Segal, T. Tota. "Lean body mass and body fat distribution in participants with chronic low back pain." *Archives of Internal Medicine* 160 (2000): 3265–69.

Volek, V. S., and E. C. Westman. "Very-low-carbohydrate weight-loss diets revisited." *Cleveland Clinic Journal of Medicine* 69 (2000): 849–62.

Wu, C. H., Y. C. Yang, W. J. Yao, et al. "Epidemiological evidence of increased bone mineral density in habitual tea drinkers." *Archives of Internal Medicine* 162 (2002): 1001–6.

Young, C. M., S. S. Scanlan, H. S. Im, et al. "Effect on body composition and other parameters in obese young men of carbohydrate level of reduction diet." *American Journal of Clinical Nutrition* 24 (1971): 290–96.

Acknowledgments

We have received generous assistance from a very select group of family, friends, and colleagues. We express our gratitude to Robert G. Bruce III; Michael Bockenek; Brittnye Bruce Bockenek, M.S.; Ashley Elizabeth Bruce; Claire Van Leuven Bruce, M.P.A.; Hugh H. Cruse, M.P.H., M.S./M.I.S.; Laura E. McIlwain Cruse, M.D.; Kimberly McIlwain, M.D.; Michael McIlwain, D.M.D.; Sunjay Daniel Trehan; Christina Yarnoz; and our graphic artist, James Russell, M.S., for his excellent artwork throughout the book.

Our agent, Denise Marcil, whose enthusiasm for a book on a holistic program for back pain motivated our creative talents.

Our editor, Deborah Brody, for appreciation of natural therapies to prevent and treat back pain.

Index

Index

About the Authors

HARRIS H. MCILWAIN, M.D., a board-certified rheumatologist, is the founder of the Tampa Medical Group. He has been researching and treating pain-related illnesses for more than twenty-five years and has published numerous articles and more than fourteen books on the subject. *Town and Country* has twice named him one of the Best Doctors in America. He lives in Temple Terrace, Florida.

DEBRA FULGHUM BRUCE, PH.D., has written more than 2,500 articles and 65 books on various health topics. She lives in Atlanta, Georgia.

Expert Advice from Harris H. McIlwain, M.D.,
and Debra Fulghum Bruce, Ph.D., for Relieving
and Preventing Pain-Related Diseases

The Fibromyalgia Handbook: A 7-Step Program
to Halt and Even Reverse Fibromyalgia
Available in Trade Paperback (ISBN 0-8050-7241-1)
The newly revised edition of this popular handbook offers hope to the
millions who suffer from the constant, severe muscle pains, relentless
fatigue, disturbed sleep, and feelings of depression associated with this
often misdiagnosed arthritis-related disease. This proven 7-step treatment
program covers the latest in medications available to lessen the symptoms
of fibromyalgia, along with exercises to reduce muscle pain and increase
strength and energy, and an expanded discussion of complementary therapies such as homeopathy, chiropractic, and herbal therapies that may
benefit sufferers.

Pain-Free Arthritis: A 7-Step Program
for Feeling Better Again
Available in Trade Paperback (ISBN 0-8050-7325-6)
Whether you suffer from the wear-and-tear pain of osteoarthritis, work-
related pain from carpal tunnel syndrome, or any other variety of arthritis,
you will find concrete, practical suggestions in this comprehensive and
effective plan. The authors distill the scientific discoveries of recent years
on the mechanisms and types of arthritis into a program that combines
exercise, nutrition, and the latest conventional and alternative therapies
to offer real relief from pain and enable you to resume an active life.

The Pain-Free Back: 6 Simple Steps to End Pain
and Reclaim Your Active Life
Available in Trade Paperback (ISBN 0-8050-7326-4)
Whether it's a short-term muscle spasm or a chronic ache, back pain strikes
four out of five adult Americans at some point in their lives. Much of this
pain can be avoided or alleviated by following the program described in
this book. The plan takes a holistic approach combining exercise, diet,
complementary and alternative medicines, lifestyle changes, and touch
therapies to strengthen the back and eliminate the factors that cause or
aggravate back pain.

Look for these titles wherever books are sold.

Owl Books